Dave & Me

Dave & Me

Life with and without my Hairy Biker

Lili Myers

Foreword by Si King

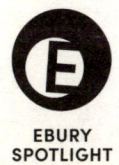

EBURY
SPOTLIGHT

EBURY SPOTLIGHT

UK | USA | Canada | Ireland | Australia
India | New Zealand | South Africa

Ebury Spotlight is part of the Penguin Random House group of companies
whose addresses can be found at global.penguinrandomhouse.com

Penguin Random House UK
One Embassy Gardens, 8 Viaduct Gardens, London SW11 7BW

penguin.co.uk
global.penguinrandomhouse.com

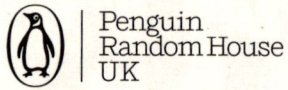 Penguin
Random House
UK

First published by Ebury Spotlight in 2025

1

Image credits:
Shutterstock (Image 1)
Milton Howard (Images 3 and 4)
Tom Baigrey (Image 11)
Jill Gibbons of Little Ninja Photography (Image 25)

The publisher and author have made every effort to credit the copyright
owners of any material that appears within, and will correct any
omissions in subsequent editions if notified.

Typeset by seagulls.net

Printed and bound in Great Britain by Clays Ltd, Elcograf S.p.A.

The authorised representative in the EEA is Penguin Random House Ireland,
Morrison Chambers, 32 Nassau Street, Dublin D02 YH68.

A CIP catalogue record for this book is available from the British Library

ISBN 9781529966541

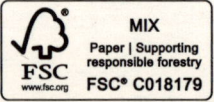 MIX
Paper | Supporting
responsible forestry
FSC® C018179

Penguin Random House is committed to a
sustainable future for our business, our readers
and our planet. This book is made from Forest
Stewardship Council® certified paper.

To my son and daughter.

Sergiu and Izabelle, I'm honoured
to be called Mum by you.

Dave and I were always in awe of you both, watching
you grow into two happy, loving and compassionate
humans. I know that you share with me many
of the feelings I express in this book, and I am
forever grateful for your support and love.

Contents

Foreword

By Si King

It is my great pleasure and honour to write the foreword for such a special book, albeit bittersweet in the writing. It's been a year since Dave passed. Even so, he doesn't stop being my best friend and is never far from my daily thoughts.

I miss his mischievous, restless spirit, his adventurous character, his curiosity, his sense of wonder about life and the world around him. His enthusiasm for the day ahead and all it had to offer was infectious and often hilarious.

Dave & Me is a glimpse into the life Dave and Lil shared together; the love they nurtured, the family that thrived and the new opportunities they embraced with gratitude and joy. They met in Sighet, Romania, Lil's hometown. Dave and I had tumbled into town while scouting for the Romanian episodes of our first TV series. We'd been on the road for some weeks at that point. Dave wanted to stay in a dodgy hotel on the outskirts, but I insisted we looked in the centre. We rocked up to reception looking like two drifters from the back woods. There on reception was Liliana. Dave stumbled over his words while chatting to Lil and I thought, *Ooooooo! There is a bit of something going on here!*

Over a drink that evening Dave said, 'Kingy, I proper fancy her!' My response was, 'You gotta be kidding! She's scary.' Taking zero notice of my opinion – quite rightly so – Dave and Lil started to chat over email and meet up when time allowed. After each event horizon had passed, Dave would say to me, 'I miss her when she's not here, Kingy.' Dave would often talk about Lil on and off screen with humour and a knowing that only comes from a deep under-standing of someone. It was a pleasure to see my best mate happy, settled and with someone he clearly loved.

This is a book Lil needed to write, a cathartic process in a step-by-step journey through the myriad of emotions that grief and loss bring. These pages are also a celebration of a love and commitment to one another that lasts beyond their painful parting.

After Dave's death we became acutely aware that so many Hairy Bikers fans were grieving too. It became very import-ant to Lili that there should be an event of some description to give everyone who loved Dave the opportunity to express their own grief, love and affection. That event was Dave Day. A day of days! 46,000 motorcycles took to the roads of the UK accompanied by 175,000 people lining the route from North London to Barrow-in-Furness, all in tribute to Lili's husband and my best mate. The fellowship and community that was felt on that day was beyond words. It was something that none of us will ever forget. I know he would have been so proud and humbled in equal measure.

Through the darkness that life often brings, Dave and Lil brought light and hope. I hope that Lil's words within this book will bring comfort to many who are going through their own loss. It is always darkest before the dawn. I know Lil now walks forwards in light and with wonderful memories of her husband and my best friend. Dave, I know, would have wished very much that it should be that way.

Love is an eternal energy that lasts. How privileged we are to be held in the embrace of love.

Until we meet again, my dear friend.

Prologue

8 June 2024

Staring at my reflection in the bathroom mirror, I'm shaking with emotion. I try taking deep breaths to calm my nerves, but the enormity of what is about to happen feels almost overwhelming.

Shall I put on mascara?

Best not. I know there will be tears later.

On his side of the shelf, I spot the bottle of his favourite Kilian perfume. I first bought it for him when he was on *Strictly Come Dancing* in 2013 and he loved it so much, he wore it from that day on.

Today I'm going to wear it for him, along with his biking jacket, helmet and goggles. In just a few hours I will be roaring along the M6 towards Barrow-in-Furness, a pillion on the back of a Harley-Davidson, followed by a procession of motorbikes riding in convoy – thousands upon thousands all making the same journey north.

A pilgrimage.

I put on my official T-shirt and his lovely twirly-tached face printed on the front smiles back at me in the mirror.

Oh, how he would have loved all this. I know he's up there laughing his snazzy socks off, thrilled to pieces that we've pulled it off.

I can hardly believe it myself. In less than three months, a casual conversation about organising a ride to honour the life of an extraordinary man has snowballed into a national event, filling my heart with pride.

From beyond the grave, he is uniting North and South – the bikers, the food lovers, the mums, dads and kids – with the convoy setting off from London in the morning, collecting riders at every stop along the 300-mile route to Barrow.

The biking community, such a tight-knit family built on the foundations of unity, mutual respect and belonging, all coming together to pay tribute to one of their own, cheered on by crowds of well-wishers gathered on motorway bridges.

And the good people of Barrow would respond in kind, opening up their homes and their hearts to meet, greet and feed perfect strangers, offering weary riders beds for the night and gardens to camp in.

I can imagine him rubbing his hands with joy at how he'd managed to bring everyone together in such a remarkable celebration of life. He put Barrow on the map and now he was bringing the country to Barrow.

The police would later confirm that 46,136 bikes took part in the ride, plus many more who were unaccounted for.

Historic.

But this would be about so much more than honouring my husband.

In a world that is shaken by hardship and where we have so much to be disheartened about, it was sublime.

A day when the world was a better place to live in.

A Dave Day.

Chapter One

How We (Don't) Talk About Death

That stuffing could raise Lazarus!

My name is Lili Myers. You probably won't know me, but I'm sure you'll know my husband, Dave.

This book is about him, our journey together and now, sadly, my journey without him. Most of all, it's a book about life and an unquenchable thirst for it. It's about the magic Mr David Myers brought into this world. His joy, his uniqueness, his burning flame!

It's a happy, meaningful story of a life like no other, my memories of Dave as a creative force and a wonderful human being and the extraordinary universe he built alongside his best friend, Simon King, as the Hairy Bikers.

I want that joy to be spread. Gosh, we need more positivity in this life and to see things in a multitude of colours, just like he did. Because of Dave, I view the world as beautiful. Who I am today is a result of my experiences with him and our 20 years together. I learned so much from him.

I learned how to be free and happy and I want to take that forward with me.

I started writing shortly after he died of cancer at the age of 66 years old on 28 February 2024, eager to get things down on the page while they were still fresh in my mind and unaltered by time. I wanted to paint the most accurate picture of who he was.

As I tidied the house we shared, touching Dave's possessions and rediscovering items I'd not thought about in a long time, I was reminded of significant moments in our life and they would inspire me to write further. At first my words were coming from acute pain, but with every line I put down, the hurt would lift a little.

The more I expressed, the lighter I felt, and it started to feel like therapy – reliving our most treasured memories has helped me process my grief.

I'd urge anyone going through hard times to try writing about those experiences – it can be a way of clearing the mind, determining what needs healing and diverting your thoughts into something positive.

As a qualified life coach and hypnotherapist, I work with people in emotional turmoil, and since losing Dave, I've been able to use that knowledge and the tools from my training to help me find a way through. In profound grief, I've known when to step back, when to step forward and when to ask for help if I've been depleted.

Now that I truly understand what it means to hold your loved one's hand as they die – the desperation, the emptiness –

I'm hoping that sharing my way of coping might help others who have not yet found a way.

That would be a privilege to me.

I would also like to open up some worthwhile conversations about death and encourage people to approach the subject with honesty and curiosity. By normalising these discussions and removing the taboo and awkwardness, we can reduce fear, strengthen connections and better support one another.

Even when we both knew the end was imminent, Dave always stubbornly refused to speak about death. His response was to shut it down or change the subject, despite my best efforts to get him to talk.

'I'm not dead yet!' he'd say, however tentatively I broached it.

That uncommunicativeness included any discussion about his funeral and, apart from his wish *not* to be cremated, he didn't leave any instructions around what he wanted me to do. It was all down to me and my imagination, which felt like a daunting prospect. This was the end of an era, but I had no clarity or guidance from him on what I should do next because that conversation never happened.

Funnily enough, years ago, long before his diagnosis, we made our wills and Dave had it written in his that he wanted the Eels track 'It's a Motherfucker' played at his funeral. Yes, really! Thankfully, he had second thoughts and later changed it – can you imagine the vicar's face if we'd carried out that particular final request ...? But that was as close as we ever came to addressing the end.

Death.

It's the only certainty in life and yet somehow we haven't perfected a way of confronting it. The mere word can unsettle us. In the West particularly, we can go out of our way to avoid talking about it, burying our heads in the sand and fearing our own mortality to the point where even the ageing process has been stigmatised. From cosmetic procedures to the chemicals we put in or on our bodies, to the way we dress and behave, all of it is designed to prioritise youth, pushing the idea of getting older into a future we'd prefer not to contemplate.

Speaking from a place of compassion and gentle observation, in Western society, we seem to have learned to cope with the nearness of death by placing some distance between ourselves and it. Our elders and the seriously ill are lovingly cared for in institutionalised facilities, but this often means that the experience of dying becomes separated from the fabric of everyday life. Death begins to feel like something far away, something we watch from a distance rather than walk through hand-in-hand.

The process of dying is therefore shrouded in mystery and, as humans, we fear what we don't know. We are not emotionally equipped to approach death in a 'matter-of-fact' way, nor are we emotionally prepared to accept it for what it is, regardless of the belief system we adopt. Death is sometimes seen not as a natural unfolding, but as a quiet defeat. This view can cause those nearing the end of life to feel as though they must slip away in solitude, rather than having their hand lovingly held in their final breath. And those left behind struggle to find closure, missing out on those sacred moments.

Dave's reluctance to address what was happening was a source of frustration to me, not least because I come from Romania, a place where people *do* talk about death, and when a person dies the whole community takes part in the rituals around their passing.

Children are included, so from a very early age they are aware of death and its finality. It's normal to keep loved ones who have passed in an open coffin in their home for three days so people can come to pay their respects and say their goodbyes. Coffins were never sinister or creepy to me and death didn't scare me because it was treated as something that was part of life. Funeral services take place in front of the local community with everybody following the coffin from the home directly to the graveyard and then assisting in the burial before heading to a commemorative dinner to mark the change in the lives of the people left behind. The family in mourning wear black clothes and black armbands for a year.

Other cultures embrace death as part of life's natural rhythm, celebrate it, ritualise it, or integrate it into daily life, all nuanced by spirituality and beliefs in afterlife. Others distance themselves from it, fear it or medicalise it. Each way has its own wisdom and challenges. But ultimately, they all reflect a deep, human need to find meaning in mortality.

My Dacian ancestors would rejoice when someone in the community was crossing over, celebrating the deceased's reunion in death with the supreme god, Zalmoxis. Traces of those beliefs can still be observed today in the northern area of Romania where I was born. In a village called Sapanta there's a 'Merry Cemetery' combining pagan rituals and symbols with Christianity. The wooden crosses are coloured in a special shade of blue and carved with funny scenes and witty lyrics about the person's life and death. When Dave and Si filmed in Romania in 2005, they visited this place and it featured in the first series of *The Hairy Bikers' Cookbook*.

Dave wasn't a very religious person, but wherever we travelled in the world, we'd make sure we paid a visit to the local church.

'Let's just go and check in,' he'd say. 'Say hello.'

My personal belief is that we keep coming back in a material form on this earth to experience and learn lessons. When the physical body expires, we remain everywhere as an energy field, part of the primordial source called God.

* * *

The first person close to me to die was my grandfather, but I was only four or five, so I don't recall much about it. Then within a very short space of time, my two little cousins who lived in the same house as us both died. The eldest was two and suffered a collapsed lung. The six-month-old baby, I believe, succumbed to cot death. I remember being in the room with their coffins, watching intently and hoping to see them start breathing again so I could be the first one to give their mother the good news that they were alive.

Understandably, death and bereavement were harder to bear the older I became and losing my grandmother when I was in my late twenties hit me hard. When we suffer loss, I believe the invisible attachment thread tying you to that person breaks, but the mind can't immediately grasp that. It doesn't compute because there are neurological pathways that are firmly formed and a large bank of memories very much embedded in your brain.

The brain likes prediction in order to keep us safe from danger and so it works hard, searching for that person, and then doesn't understand why it can't find them. Those connections don't dissolve when the object of our emotional attachment is separated from us – we still crave that connection and ache when we can't find it. It takes time to alter the bond and change the structures – indeed, it took me about three years after my grandmother's death to break the pattern of searching for her in the house.

The magnitude of losing your life partner is on a different level because it completely shatters the balance built up from years of trust, work, commitment and love. In the chaos that ensues, we lose our identity and keep trying to find elements of familiarity. The consistency we crave is no longer there, although we constantly seek it and search for anything related to them – a song, a place, a jumper that once hugged their body – hoping it might give us back a feeling, a smell, a sensation that will make us feel better.

That search can feel desperate.

I tried it many times, finding Dave. In a shirt, in food, in my travels, in my dreams. Five months after his death I impulsively drove my car alone from my home in the UK, taking a ferry across the Channel and then driving through France, Belgium, Germany, Austria, Hungary and Romania, into the village of Viscri where Dave and Si had filmed nearly 20 years earlier, simply for its connections with him. I drove through the heart of that village, searching for traces of Dave, knowing how much he loved the place and remembering his tales of Sarah and her chicken noodle soup. After roaming around aimlessly I left disappointed, not having found any feelings there nor anything to remind me of him.

And that's when I realised that a place in this material space is not what will bring me Dave's presence, smell or spirit. It's completely natural to try to latch on to everything we can in an attempt to reconnect, but to heal and move forward we need to untie and refocus. That means understanding the impact our lost loved ones had on our lives, the lessons we learned from them, the gifts they bestowed, and then taking all of that with us.

I thought of Dave's final moments when I was at his bedside, telling him how much I loved him and that if he needed to go, I would be all right. By then he was heavily sedated, seemingly between worlds and hadn't been responsive for a number of days, but all of a sudden he replied, 'I'm not going anywhere!'

That was Dave.

It makes me smile now because, of course, he was quite right. He's not gone. He's still everywhere, in every aspect of my life, my home and my mind.

The Medallion

24 May 2024

It's early morning and I'm taking my dog, Teddy, out for a walk. The spring sun is beginning to rise and the air is crisp, bringing my senses back to life after another broken night's sleep. The night-times are difficult. It's been three months since Dave died and while the days are busy enough for me to push my thoughts and feelings aside, at night I'm alone with nowhere to hide.

That's when everything I've been avoiding comes back to bite and I toss and turn the what-ifs over and over, my head spinning, pushing me to the brink of exhaustion … but never quite tipping me over the edge into a deep sleep. My poor body is so tired. I can't find peace. Every time I feel the pain ease a little and my balance doesn't seem quite so off-kilter, something comes out of nowhere to obliterate the stillness. A smell, a picture, something he touched, a song he loved, a feather landing at my feet.

And it digs deep, like a blade.

Grief occupies the mind, body and spirit, taking its time to develop, settle and resolve. I guess I need to give it time. A lot of time. An eternity, maybe.

But today my mood is good as an excitable Teddy and I march through the Staffordshire countryside – my beautiful, madcap rescue dog is putting a smile on my face as he pulls on the lead, forcing me to keep up. We take the usual path across the lawn, following the trail around the lake, Teddy stopping for his habitual sniff in the bushes. He runs circles round the trees, chases squirrels and jumps at the geese, causing them to collectively honk and flap their wings before skimming across the water to escape him.

I love Teddy for what he does for me every day. For loving me unconditionally when I don't know how to love myself. I almost feel sorry for him having to put up with me as I struggle to find a new way to live.

Teddy came to us quite unexpectedly.

Having sadly lost two beloved dogs during the pandemic, Dave and I had been discussing adopting another. Our friend Tara McDonald oversaw the makeup department for the Netflix series *Wednesday* and while filming in Bucharest, Romania, one of her colleagues had found an abandoned pup on a skip near the set. He was the sole survivor of a litter of five and when Tara posted about him on Facebook, both Dave and I had the same thought. Admittedly, we were a tad hungover after a night on the vino and jumped in almost without thinking to offer this little mite a home.

The wheels were set in motion and two months later, having sorted all the paperwork, Teddy became part of our family. His arrival ended up coinciding with Dave being diagnosed with cancer and although Teddy felt like a blessing for me, Dave used to say, 'That dog will live longer than me ...' Months later when we bumped into Tara and her husband, Luke Morley, at an event, Dave teased her, 'It's all your fault!'

Ha! The memories that come up ...

I start to head home, looking forward to a well-earned cup of coffee and a sit down with my sewing. Teddy's tail is wagging with delight and all seems calm and peaceful on this beautiful but otherwise unremarkable day.

It's when I arrive back that I find it.

Sitting on the first of the stairs up to the house is a little silver medallion, glinting in the sunlight. I pick it up and the inscription causes my heart to jolt and my knees to buckle.

If i had my life to live all over again
i would find you sooner
so i could love you longer

HOW? Where I live is quite remote; there are no passers-by, no dog walkers and no public path, but this small silver disc has found its way into my world. I flip it over and feel it resting in my palm for a few moments and then I clutch it tightly, swallowed from head to toe by a hot wave of grief.

My mind is scrambling to find an explanation. I can't come up with one. I consider the possibility that it's all a mere coincidence with no personal connotation and that it just so happened to fall from someone's pocket. On my stairs. I almost manage to convince myself this is no sign. Of course it's not a message from across time and space! How could it be? It's a trivial item with no significance at all.

And yet …

Call me foolish, but even if conventional wisdom dictates that this message can't have transcended two worlds, I want to hold on to what the words represent. Because the truth is I *do* wish I'd met him a lot earlier in my life and I *do* wish I'd had more time to feel loved by him and to make him see how much happiness he brought into my world.

Into this *whole* world.

I wish I had the power to bottle up his energy and exuberance, his zest for life and for living, his laughter and playfulness, his sparkle and his brilliance. I wish he'd had the chance to know how special he was and what an impact his life had on so many others.

Dave and I were lucky to have 20 years of shared dreams. Two decades of adventure and togetherness and love and explosion and colour. Our first dance at our wedding in 2011 was 'Rock You Like a Hurricane' by Scorpions and, my goodness, that was exactly our life. It was 100 miles an hour – maybe more! – but what a beautiful ride it was.

He gave me those years of his life and I gave him mine. What we were denied – the future we had planned – is too painful to contemplate just now.

I see older couples playing with their grandchildren in the park and I know we will never have that time together. How he would have loved to have shared moments like those. And what a fantastic grandad he would have been. How can I live in a future that was supposed to be enjoyed together and with a pain that can't be healed, only carried?

I'm still coming to terms with the fact that however much I tried, it wasn't in my power to fix Dave. There have been many tears and lingering doubts over whether I did enough, and in the chaos that came after his death, I turned against myself for not having had the power to save him. For having missed signs that might have helped an earlier diagnosis or given a better outcome. For losing my temper in moments when I was so frightened I had no clue how to react. For my moments of anger when we could have had peace. For the glimpses of happiness that we missed. For living, when he was denied that privilege.

Untangling those thoughts and feelings will take time, but I don't want my pain to define me, so I have to let go and learn to fill all the space Dave has left with worthy things, knowing that he's always going to be the best part of me.

That is my grieving process.

I steady myself and open the front door. Teddy bounds into the house, keen to receive his post-walk doggie treat and fresh bowl of water. I head into my office and gently place the mysterious medallion on the desk where I will be able to see it every day. Wherever it came from, I know I will keep it forever.

I tell myself that it didn't matter how much I loved him or how much he wanted to live, it wasn't going to happen and so the 'why' questions are pointless. 'Why' is a vicious circle. The longer you stay in the 'why' zone, the more prolonged the grief and the more complicated it becomes, so I'm going to try instead to ask different questions and focus on the wonderful 20 years Dave gave me.

But I will always wish that we'd met earlier in life.

I wish.

I wish.

Chapter Two

A Bit About Me

Fluffier than a chick that's come out of a tumble drier!

Dave used to say to me, 'Lil, what are the odds of a boy from a council house on a backstreet in Barrow-in-Furness, getting to do the things I do? I'll tell you what: less than winning the lottery!'

We never won a lottery, but we felt we beat the odds by meeting each other in the first place and going on to live a life full of fun, connection, friendship and fabulous food. We were so *lucky* to find each other and to bring our worlds together. Because really, what *are* the chances that two people from such different backgrounds, such different countries and with such different experiences of life, would meet and fall so deeply in love?

Allow me to tell you a little about where I come from and you'll see what I mean. I was born Liliana Boroica and I grew up in Sighet, a small, quiet town in the north of Romania. My family struggled, like many others living under communist rule, but they did the best they could in difficult circumstances to offer my sister and me a good home.

In 1966, the same year as my birth, a law was passed making abortion illegal unless the woman already had four living children. The legislation, aimed at boosting Romania's low birth rates, was known as Decree 770 and so my generation were dubbed 'the decree children'.

The tragedies that followed were numerous and unspeakably sad, the situation exacerbated by a total lack of any form of sex education or the availability of contraceptive advice. It was illegal to terminate a pregnancy but also frowned upon to be a single mother. Women in abusive relationships, those unable to financially afford a child or who had any other reason not to keep a pregnancy were trapped between two terrible scenarios. Many were forced into backstreet abortions and thousands bled to death.

Unwanted children were given up or taken away and put into state-run orphanages where institutional abuse was rife and unchecked, and there are conservative estimates of 100,000 abandoned babies.

The first images to emerge in the Western media about Romania following the fall of the communist dictatorship in December 1989 were of the squalid orphanages and malnourished children – they shocked the world and the stories behind those pictures reflected the politics of the time. There were many heart-breaking stories; some remain untold and hidden because they were seen as shameful secrets.

Dave and Me

The brutal secret police – the Securitate – were all-knowing and all-powerful. In my early thirties I worked as a curator in a museum that had been a communist prison. From 1945 until the seventies, the political and intellectual elites of the country had been imprisoned and killed there by the emerging dictatorship. Working there connected me with thousands of people who had stories of atrocious abuse suffered under the Securitate oppression, many for no other fault than having the same surname as a political prisoner. Or being in the wrong place at the wrong time. Others, very bravely, had tried to defy the system and change things ...

But there is so much more to my homeland than the traumas of the past, and the Romania I love and cherish is beautiful, rich in cultural heritage and possesses a strength of spirit that survived centuries of turmoil.

Dave always loved my country, its people and traditions – there are wonderful places to visit throughout – not just Bran Castle, made famous by Bram Stoker's *Dracula* and which so many tourists make a beeline for. Geographically, the Carpathian Mountains are the spinal column of Romania, crossing the land horizontally and then bending vertically towards the north. The flat lands to the south were once considered the wheat fields of Europe, and the Danube River borders the south of the country then flows towards the east into the Black Sea, forming a beautiful delta – now a protected area as many species of animals find it a haven. Northeast of the Carpathians is Moldavia, with its historical painted churches, while Transylvania is to the northwest.

In my opinion, the north (where I am from) is the best! I know, I'm biased and I'm sure many of you feel the same about the places you are connected to. Maramureș in northern Transylvania is the county I was born in. It's mostly mountains, with a couple of rivers between summits reaching over 3,000 metres. On old maps dating from the sixteenth century, those mountains were known as *Monster Lupii* or 'Mountains of the Wolves' and it is still true today that wolves roam freely up there.

I remember holidays spent in the countryside with my paternal grandparents and long winter nights listening to the wolves howling in the distance. Today the territory remains very much wild, with deep forests and a rich flora and fauna.

In 1920, after the First World War and following a long period of political upheaval, the Treaty of Trianon established Romania's new northern border on the Tisza River, splitting Maramureș. One third stayed in the territory that became part of the newly formed Czechoslovakia and which now belongs to Ukraine.

I grew up right by that river, able to see activity and life on the other side, but never allowed to cross it. My maternal grandmother was born on the opposite bank in a village called Biserica Alba and when I was growing up, we could not get in touch with or meet family left across the water.

The population of northern Romania was of Thracian origin – history refers to them as Free Geto-Dacian people because they avoided Roman rule during the conquests of the early centuries of the first millennium. However, throughout history the land has had to withstand many wars and much devastation along with vast change and migration.

Over the centuries, the population has embraced an ancient culture that blends pagan elements with Christianity. Wood has been the main construction material and the wooden churches with their tall, steep spires have long become an emblem of that territory. The oldest wooden church still in use, named the Church on the Hill, dates to the seventeenth century – its walls feature the original murals.

Along the villages on the Iza Valley, the river that shapes the Maramureş depression, there are wooden gates carved with pagan symbols such as the sun and moon, rope as a blend of positive and negative, and the tree of life. The more ornate, the richer the family.

Folklore is well kept and well loved, and dances, songs, fairy tales, poems and costumes represent a long-established identity. Summers there are sunny and idyllic with abundant vegetation and rural life has not changed much with time – people still mow their meadows with scythes, plough the land with horses or oxen and use the moon phases and seasons to plan their crops and lives.

Rituals such as lighting beacons on hilltops in the night of Sanziene after the summer solstice, chanting spells for wealth, finding love, healthy crops or protecting the livestock, have evolved into local events and festivals, and are now a tourist attraction.

The higher summits are covered in thick forest and one tradition still adhered to is herding the sheep up to the higher pastures in spring and keeping them in designated areas called *stână* where they are cared for by the shepherds for the whole summer. When the greenery turns to autumnal copper shades, they all return down to the villages.

In winter, women set up looms in their front rooms, weaving the wool they spin and dye in colourful patterns, or hand-embroidering dowry for their daughters and hanging their creations on wooden shelves for everybody to admire.

The houses are a magical display of colour and craft.

* * *

My family were hardworking, but we never had holidays, parties or rewards. I don't think my parents ever experienced true happiness unless it was related to their two daughters – myself and my little sister, Mirela. I always called their cohort the sacrificial generation: war babies and then communist doctrine adults.

My mum and dad married after a very short courtship and for the first four years of my childhood, we all lived in my maternal grandmother's home on the edge of a small town. It was a tiny council house with a corridor that served as a kitchen, dining room and my grandparents' bedroom. My grandfather was ill and unable to walk, and I only remember him as a white-haired man who was always lying down. On either side of the corridor were two small rooms, one occupied by the four of us and the other by my uncle's family and their two baby boys.

My grandma gave us a small patch of her vegetable garden where my dad, Vasile, built our family home himself in his spare time while also working a full-time job. None of us had leisurely weekends – everyone would have to pitch in with whatever was happening on the building site, whether that was painting, carrying bricks or digging holes.

I was a teenager by the time the house was finished and the building mess settled. After that, my father started to take jobs for the neighbours on our street, all in his free time. He was a master at soldering and would make metallic gates, fences and greenhouses.

Dad was employed all his active life as the leader of a team in a factory producing nuts and bolts for heavy industry. Sometimes as a child I'd visit him at work to find him under a big metal lathe, his hands blackened with dirt and his clothes smelling of burnt oils. He was a hero to many, with apprentices under his care and the whole production line depending on him. He'd bring home paperwork to figure out the rotas and calculate wages and would give me a spare sheet to write my own table with made-up employee names. I loved those hours I got to spend with him even though his attention was not entirely mine.

He was always working, never free.

My mum, Veronica, was the youngest daughter of my grandmother's eight surviving children, and very beautiful as a young woman, I've been told. She was just 17 when she married, 18 when I was born and 19 when my sister came along. We were lucky that she could stay home with us in our early years but she later worked shifts at the same factory as my father. Apart from her cousin Marioara, I don't remember her having friends or socialising outside the house or going anywhere without my dad, who was jealous and protective.

Dad was the one who made most of the decisions while Mum was the quiet, enduring one. She had to be because the ugly matter of alcohol always loomed large, as it did with many families in that time and place. There were no forms of entertainment, joy or release, except the escape that alcohol – cheap and readily available – provided. My father was solid and dependable when he was sober, but around paydays, he became a different person.

And it was my mum who had to bear the aggression, abuse, pain, shame and all the troubles of an overworked man. Those days were horrible and messy and my mum battled depression … They loved each other and they loved us – that was very clear to us children – although the word 'love' was never used in front of us, or towards us. It was not usual to express or discuss your feelings like that.

Money was always tight and I'd often walk to school with tarnished shoes, a broken backpack or wearing old clothes.

Water had to be manually pumped from the garden and I'd do my homework by candlelight to save on electricity. My grandmother would say: 'Money is round and has to roll ...' Well, it rolled out of our hands as soon as the salary was paid. Everyone worked for the state in one form or another and salaries barely stretched from one payday to the next. This uneasy relationship with money was something that followed me throughout my life and took a long time to get over.

My sister and I, like most of the kids in those days, grew up queuing. Every day we would have to line up for milk and bread, and once a month we'd be given tickets for cooking oil, a kilo of sugar and one of flour. Queuing was essential because the stock was limited and people often ended up not having their rations because of shortages in supply.

Occasionally we could queue for a kilo of salami or sausage and once or twice a year we'd be lucky to get some fresh meat. Before Christmas it was two oranges per head and a pack of butter. Toilet paper and soap were a luxury we'd rarely see and if you wanted to buy clothes, you'd struggle to find anything of quality in the shops. Everything Romania produced during those years was meant to be exported. We were left with the scraps.

There was a level of acceptance though, because we didn't know life could be better and austerity taught us from childhood to make do with what was available. Control, censorship and communist propaganda were everywhere and you learned from a very early age that if you wanted to stay out of bother, you kept your mouth shut. The authoritarian militia ruled by fear and could make anyone disappear. We were like little flies they could flick away and get rid of, and we all knew of people captured, killed or imprisoned for supposedly stepping out of line.

A friend of mine, Valy, used to play guitar and by some miracle he'd managed to obtain some Beatles music on a cassette. He'd also let his hair grow. One day he was stopped on the street by two officers and asked, 'Hey, you tramp, what's with this hair of yours? You know you're not allowed long hair!'

Valy timidly replied, 'I admire John Lennon and I want to be like him.'

'You're coming with us. And we'll get our hands on that Lennon guy as well!'

They forced him to cut his hair.

Western society was described to us as corrupt, depraved, anarchist. The borders were closed to us and we didn't have passports or any knowledge of what was happening in the rest of the world. We only had two hours of television on weekdays, just enough for a news bulletin and a Soviet movie about war, armies and defeated Germans. However, we used to look forward to Thursday nights because there would be an extra half an hour of music on TV – two or three songs from foreign singers and then the rest of the time given to young Romanian artists.

One Thursday, the programme stopped suddenly with a message about 'technical problems'. Much later we discovered it had been because one of the female singers was wearing a skirt above the knee, which was deemed too short by the president's wife, who interrupted the show and cut it. We never got those Thursday nights of music back.

There were outlets, but they came with risk. In the eighties, Radio Free Europe would broadcast in Romanian at midnight each night from Munich. They featured letters sent in by dissidents or families of people under political arrest; testimonies of the reality in oppressed Romania which described the hardship, the tyranny and everything else. Many of us managed to tune in but it was illegal to listen and if we'd been caught it would have meant big trouble. After the letters there was about an hour of Western music and I'd hear the British DJ Johnnie Walker broadcasting from London, which felt revolutionary.

What Johnnie Walker's voice represented for us was modernity, the West and a portal to a different world.

It allowed us to dream.

* * *

When I was about eight, my young English language teacher gave me the address of a girl in the UK called Claire, thinking we could be penpals. I wrote Claire a letter in my very limited English and a few weeks later I received a reply. I was ecstatic to have made such a connection! She even sent me her photo!

She was a similar age to me with red curly hair and a lovely smiling face. I wrote back to her but didn't have a photo of myself to send. I never got a reply that time and always thought Claire must be upset with me for not sending her my photo. Years later my mum told me the truth. My letter had been intercepted and my parents had been summoned to the Securitate and questioned about why their daughter was in touch with foreign forces. Imagine doing that to an eight-year-old girl. That was the level of control they had.

I was always a bright student. I had a good memory and was very creative, but I was also serious for my age – I never played at school and I don't remember laughing too much either. I wouldn't say I was a leader, but certainly I was a watcher. An observer.

I could stick up for myself, though. There was a competition in my class to get the highest marks at the end of the school year, and one time I ended up in a physical fight with a boy who was unhappy at coming second. I was left with a fistful of his hair in my hand while he was holding the ripped collar of my uniform in his. A few years on, when we were in our late teens, the same boy tried to date me and it was a big fat 'no' from me, remembering our previous scuffle. I was not one to get bullied or soften my guard.

I loved books, although censorship meant what we had available was limited and I'd read with a torch under the covers at night so as not to wake my grandma, who slept in the same room. Books were my escape and fuelled my imagination. I was blessed to live with my grandmother because she was quite a character. She moved in with us into the house my father built after the death of my grandfather and her own story is worthy of a novel. It cuts across countries, borders, two world wars, an imprisoned husband who was deported to Siberia, lost children, collectivisation and poverty.

She gave birth to ten children amid all this.

My grandma was illiterate but she had a wealth of knowledge and was a model of stoicism – I think she had to be to survive everything she did. She would tell us stories about her experiences and it all seemed surreal to us as kids. I wish I'd paid more attention to those stories, because now there's no actual testimony left, no documents or written proof of that extraordinary past.

I'm not sure how warm and loving she could have been with her own kids due to the harsh context of their lives, but with Mirela and me she was strict and wise and always there. I learned to cook by watching her and there's a funny story that Dave loved. When teaching me how to use the rolling pin, she used to tell me, 'Be careful, girl, if you don't roll it properly your man will take the rolling pin and beat you up!' Every time Dave made pasta, he'd ask me to roll it and tell him that story and he'd roar with laughter.

* * *

My first job after leaving school was in a factory that mass-produced clothing for Western Europe. Years later, when I told Dave about it, he referred to it as a 'sweatshop'

– I'd never thought of it like that, but realised that's exactly what it was.

One day, a few militia officers gathered all of us around a poor man they'd brought in wearing handcuffs. They told us he had been arrested and tried for not having a job and now he was being made an example of. I don't know what happened to him next. I dread to think.

The revolution of December 1989, the execution of Ceaușescu and the fall of communism made space for a plethora of things we hadn't experienced before. People were able to travel abroad and learn about other ways of life. The market was flooded with all sorts of new products and produce and we finally understood that it was possible to live without the fear of being punished for speaking our minds.

By the time I went back to complete my education, I had become a mother. I gained a degree in tourism and hotel management and took a job managing a small hotel while raising my son and daughter, Sergiu and Izabelle. I also worked as an associate lecturer in one of the northern universities, teaching tourism and small-business management to groups of future B&B owners and administrators which I found very rewarding. I loved what I did for a living, although it meant time with my kids was limited and I had none at all for myself.

It dawned on me that I'd replicated exactly what my parents had done when I was a child. Work, work, work, just to make sure the family stayed afloat. History repeating itself, unhealthy patterns rolling into the next generation.

Dave and Me

Although I'd always worked hard, the money I earned was never enough for anything but survival. I remember one time when I was pregnant with my daughter and walking home from work, I saw apples in the window of a grocery shop. I didn't have the money for a kilo, so bought just one and ate it on my way home, only to feel incredibly ashamed for not having saved it for my son who was four years old.

I'd got married in 1988 to the father of my children, Ioan. We liked each other and at the time it felt right to settle down and start a family, just as all our friends were doing. We were so happy to welcome Sergiu and Iza, and for a while we managed well. But times changed with communism gone and, as a new way of life evolved, both Ioan and I realised that we had different ways of seeing the world.

Eventually I outgrew a relationship where we kept doing the same things over and over again, hoping for different results. Things were not right and the cracks were showing. I never wanted the children to feel anything except stability, but neither did I want them to grow up thinking that being over-worked, unhappy and grumpy was normal. I lost friendships over the decision to divorce and that hurt. In my wider family, divorce was frowned upon and my father stopped talking to me altogether. My mother told me numerous times to think of her and all her suffering over the years with my father and how she'd put up with it to keep the family together.

That only made me more determined to break away, because I could remember only too well the misery the two of them went through – I wanted the cycle of suffering to stop with my generation and not be passed on to the next.

It took me a long time to fully open up to Dave about my past. I hadn't grown up talking about my feelings; we'd been expected to go through life without complaining. No money for food? Get on with it. Man up, don't cry or show weakness and keep your worries to yourself. The patterns we learn as children are ingrained in our brains and behaviours, and unless we understand the mechanics of that, changing is not easy. Even now when I see a police officer, I freeze in fear because that was my instinctive reaction as a child.

Dave was so free and I loved that about him. We had no money when we first got together – the Hairy Bikers were in their infancy and yet to bring about any financial security – but he was a maestro at transforming every situation into something golden.

I was limited in that sense because I came from a place where we'd been taught to be robots, not to excel or to be different. Dave was the one who encouraged me to try new things, however outrageous they seemed to me!

Jumping on the handlebars of a motorbike being driven on a vertical velodrome dubbed the Wall of Death?

'Go for it, Lil!' he laughed.

Yeah … I passed on that one.

But I learned from him to go for things, to give them my best shot, to feel the fear and the doubt but to go ahead and do it anyway! Although on paper it looked like Dave and

I were a million miles apart, we found common ground in much of our outlook. Because of our childhoods – both difficult for different reasons – we didn't want to waste any time. We were hellbent on making the most of everything, having come such a long way.

Such a long way.

Because now, here's a thing.

The first New Year's Eve I spent in the UK having moved to be with Dave in September 2007, he and I went to the New Forest in Hampshire where one of the chefs he worked with had a place. Also partying away that night was Johnnie Walker and his wife Tiggy, which knocked me for six in the best possible way.

Johnnie and I were introduced and I told him the story of me and my friends listening to him illegally during the eighties and how much his broadcasts had meant to us. He'd never known that his shows were repeated on Radio Free Europe and was astonished and delighted to hear this. I'm so glad I had the opportunity to tell him.

Isn't life funny? And oh so very magical.

The Shirt

/ June 2024

For the umpteenth time in recent months, I'm trying to empty the knick-knack-filled mirrored drawers on Dave's side of the bed. Every time I've tried, I've failed to complete the task. Each little thing I touch reminds me of a moment, an experience, a place, and I've not been able to bring myself to move any of it. Anchors to a past that meant so much.

Dave and I were both hoarders. Big time! Old concert tickets, business cards, ancient menus from restaurants that probably no longer exist, maps of towns, leaflets for events long passed, ripped-out recipe pages from magazines, boarding passes for flights, small containers that had lost their contents ... all chucked into these drawers with the intention that one day we'd go through them.

Having these items from our collective history made us feel safe, grounded to our past and shared points of reference. A link to happy moments – so many of them – and what I'm trying to do now feels impossible amid an overload of emotions.

Our bedroom here is quite small – it was the convenience of having it on the ground floor that made us choose it from the others. When we moved into this house, Dave was suffering severe neuropathy as a side effect of the cancer treatment and was unable to climb stairs, so the sensible solution was to take the bedroom with the easiest access. And when I say 'small', it's not exactly poky. There's plenty of room for these side tables, a chest of drawers and space around the bed to reach the bathroom with ease.

Plenty of room too for pain and tears, for dreams and hopes, and for loss.

To give myself a moment's respite, I turn my head away from the drawers and my eyes fall on the bedroom door, where Dave's shirt is hanging on a hook. I haven't moved it, it's right there in the place he left it. He loved that soft flannel shirt with its black-and-white plaid print, the last one he ever ordered for himself online. It still smells of his perfume; I only need to look at it to catch the scent.

My mind jumps back in time to when I first visited him in Barrow in 2006. That March was particularly cold and the weather on Roa Island where he lived was damp and windy, so Dave lent me one of his many plaid shirts. It was so huge I could wrap it twice around my body and I remember clearly how soft and cosy it was and how the traces of his perfume on the fabric made me feel comforted.

I made a point of wearing that shirt every day during my two-week visit and when I left to return to Romania, I hung it on a hook on the bedroom door. Over the following weeks and months during our long-distance phone conversations, Dave would sit on the side of the bed I'd slept in, looking at the shirt I'd left hanging and he'd say, 'I just look at it, I won't disturb it, it's where you left it and that's where you'll find it when you come back.' I did go back and, sure enough, I found the shirt untouched. I wore it again.

And now here I am, looking at this shirt of Dave's which I daren't move in case I break a spell that was cast many years ago, a silent agreement between shirts and the bedroom doors they were hung on, waiting for someone to come back.

Only this time I must accept the reality that he won't be returning to wear it again.

I sit with my emotions, acknowledging their existence and allowing myself to feel them. As humans we are wired to do whatever we can to avoid having to 'hug the cactus'. We steer clear of facing the storm head on, hoping that by some miracle it will pass. Nietzsche said, 'You must have chaos within you to give birth to a dancing star,' meaning the challenges of life can uncover new strength and lead to growth. As intense as it is, feeling those emotions, recognising their nuances and dancing rather than fighting with them is what is going to lead to acceptance and learning to move forward.

There are days when that seems to be easier, not because the pain has ceased – it's still very much present and alive – but because I've become stronger at carrying it with me. Right now though, I feel like that shirt on the bedroom door, hanging by one hook, waiting. Without a body to fill it, there's no shape to it, no identity, just an empty shell.

The emptiness hurts but at the same time, I don't want to let it go because that's what is connecting me to him. If I let this pain go, I might lose him again. If I don't talk about him or to him, he will no longer have a voice. It actually feels like I've lost Dave repeatedly and each time it hurts in a different way.

I lost him a little bit every day as the illness advanced, he was undisturbed by all the medication he was given. I lost him when we were told the treatment was not working and I could see in his eyes that he was giving up. I lost him when he could no longer eat or move, and when he drew his last breath, holding my hand. I lost him when I had to tell my mum he'd passed, and then again when we had to make the news known to the public. I lost him when I had to say goodbye, watching his remains laid to rest. I lose him every time I have to tell someone that my husband died. And I lose him each morning I wake up and turn to see his shape not there in the bed next to me.

I go back to the drawer, determined to make a start. The black bin bag lies on the floor, ready to claim its victims. It's time. I've got to learn to live so I can honour his life free of this clutter.

As I begin the cleaning and cleansing process, I know that with every memory I discard into that black bag, I'm losing another piece of him.

Chapter Three

Dave

*My mam crimped the
pie's edge with her false teeth*

Where do I even begin? How can I possibly encapsulate in a single chapter the years of a man who lived so completely and experienced more in one lifetime than most could cram into ten?

People knew Dave Myers as the fun-loving TV star who threw himself into everything he did with gusto, a big smile and an open heart. They'd say he was generous to a fault, full of mischief and hugely popular.

And he was all of that.

But the truth is, Dave had a tremendously difficult start in life and went on to suffer a great deal of tragedy and affliction as an adult. Part of what made him such an exceptional person was that he never allowed any of those many misfortunes to hold him back. Despite the rotten hands he was dealt, he remained decent and honourable, inspired and inspiring, and always so full of gratitude for what he had.

He built his life by trusting in his capabilities, never thinking for one minute that he would fail. Even when things did not seem to go his way, he found the silver lining and the lesson and he'd start afresh. Nothing fazed him and I found his sense of freedom intoxicating. My husband. A straightforward, honest man who loved clarity and couldn't stand chaos.

Dave covered a lot of his early life experiences in *Blood, Sweat and Tyres*, the autobiography he co-wrote in 2015 together with Si, and I'm wary about repeating too much of that here. However, I would like to share some untold stories and important details that I feel paint a picture of the boy Dave was, the man he became and the events that shaped him.

David James Myers was born in Barrow-in-Furness to Margaret and Jim Myers on 8 September 1957, delighting his parents when a suspected ovarian cyst turned out instead to be a much-wanted baby boy.

The family lived in a small two-up, two-down terraced house on Devon Street in the town and young David was an inquisitive and energetic child who kept Margaret and Jim on their toes with his relentless curiosity. He once told me the story of how, as a six-year-old, he spilled some red tile paint on the living room carpet and decided that the only solution was to tip the remainder of the tin out and paint the rest of the floor. He thought it might be a nice surprise for his parents …

I can only imagine the horror on his poor mother's face as she laid eyes on his handiwork – she mustn't have known whether to laugh, get on her knees and scrub or to be angry at a catastrophe that would eat into the family food budget, already stretched to the max.

Then there was the tale of him building an aeroplane out of a cardboard box and attempting to take off from the Myers' six-foot-high back wall, only to plummet to the ground, breaking both his thumbs in the process. Unperturbed, as his father brought him home from hospital with his hands in casts, Dave revealed grand plans to build a boat next, adding that he'd need some tools ...

'Son, that's not a wise thing to do ...' came the reply from a weary Jim who, understandably, immediately put his toolbox under lock and key.

His parents, who were both widowed when they met, had Dave late in life – Margaret was 41 and Jim 55 – and he had one much older brother, Kenneth, from his dad's first marriage. Dave spoke very little about Kenneth, and for reasons I never really got to know, the connection between the brothers wasn't there. It may have had something to do with the fact that there were more than 30 years between them and Kenneth had his own family by the time Dave was born.

Kenneth died quite young, so I never got to meet him, although I have met his daughters – Dave's nieces – and I'm pleased to say we are in touch occasionally. We have been very close with the family of his cousin Les Myers – wonderful people who made me feel welcome from the beginning.

Dave loved his parents very much, especially his dad, who retired as foreman of the local paper mill when Dave was nine and therefore had a lot of time for his son. Jim Myers was a chain smoker and although money was always tight, Dave noted that 'there was always enough for my dad's fags'. He vividly remembered Jim's nicotine-stained fingers trying to knot a fishing line to the hook – he inherited his love of fishing from his father, as well as 'the Myers nose' as Dave used to say.

His passion for motorbikes came from his dad, too. Jim had a couple of bikes (a BSA Bantam and a Norton Dominator) when Dave was little and I think it was the freedom biking gave them and the magic of being with his dad that got him smitten.

Margaret Myers fell ill with multiple sclerosis when Dave was only eight and as much as he loved his mum, many of his memories of her were attached to that wretched health battle over the next 16 years. There were, however, a few things he lovingly remembered and appreciated about his mum – always 'Mam' to Dave – namely her humour and quick wit, which he inherited from her in abundance.

'My mam was a poet, you know?' he'd tell me when reminiscing about Margaret's advice or her funny, wise words.

It was by watching her in the kitchen that Dave first learned to cook. When she was still fit and well, Margaret would bake bread, pies, scones and cakes. She made her own bramble jelly from blackberries picked by Dave and she'd serve up hearty roast chicken dinners with all the trimmings. He once told me that his mum used her dentures to seal pies in their dish before baking them. I suspect it was a bit of a myth, but imagine that!

As his mum's health and mobility declined, Dave took on the role of chef in the house, but it was never a chore to him because he found food fascinating and likened cooking to 'being let loose in the science class ... without the teacher there to spoil the fun!' I like to picture him as a young boy following the recipes for stews, pies and soups from his mother's cookbooks and experimenting with different ingredients to make those dishes his own – not knowing that this exciting new hobby was setting the stage for what was to come much later.

Life was challenging, though. Within a year of Margaret's diagnosis, she was in a wheelchair and, in time, became physically and mentally ravaged by illness and medication. Dave and his dad were her full-time carers which was an immense responsibility for a boy not yet ten.

Social services eventually moved them to a ground-floor flat on a new council estate in Barrow and the family lived hand-to-mouth, surviving on Jim's pension money. There were many other challenges to contend with, but Dave found escape in music and painting, two more lifelong loves alongside bikes and food.

His talent for drawing and painting caught the attention of his art teacher at Barrow-in-Furness Grammar School for Boys, Mr Eaton, who became a beacon of light for Dave during the toughest of times. Mr Eaton arranged trips to art galleries and instilled in Dave his obsession with the Pre-Raphaelite Brotherhood which, forty-odd years later, would be his specialist subject for a winning turn on *Celebrity Mastermind*.

Thanks to Mr Eaton, Dave started to believe in himself, passing all 11 O-levels and staying on for sixth form to study Art, History, English and General Studies at A level. It was Mr Eaton too, who encouraged him to consider applying to university. By 1977, Dave Myers, this working-class lad who had faced so much adversity in his young life, was starting a degree in Fine Art at London's prestigious Goldsmiths University. Three hundred miles and a world away from Barrow.

* * *

Not many people know that Dave Myers, the Hairy Biker, was bald from childhood until his forties. At a very young age he began to suffer with alopecia which made things extremely difficult for him, especially in school where he was already singled out for being a 'poor kid' thanks to his free meal tokens. He was a target for the bullies and those days were miserable for Dave, sapping his confidence and spirit.

The alopecia developed at around the same time Margaret became ill and I know he often wondered if the pressure and angst at home might have been a contributing factor to his hair loss. And there was something else that emerged much later in December 1998 when he was in his early forties and collapsed while working on a film set in Luxembourg. A German hospital scan revealed an arachnoid cyst on the left side of his brain which was thought to have been there since childhood because Dave's brain had grown around it.

Against advice from doctors and friends, he travelled in his van (driven by a colleague), back to his home in Aberdeenshire where he was admitted to the Royal Infirmary for an operation to install a shunt to relieve the pressure, plus drains to remove the fluid from the cyst itself. Thankfully, the surgery was a success and Dave was discharged just five days later on Christmas Eve, but his recovery took some unexpected turns.

Not long after his op, Dave's hair started to grow in dark and healthy curls. I'm not medically trained and so this is just a hunch, but perhaps that cyst sitting undetected had been pressing on a certain part of the brain … and maybe a combination of that and the stress of caring for his mum had triggered the alopecia in the first place? We'll never know for sure, but it makes sense to me.

I could still feel the shunt on the left side of Dave's head when I met him seven years later, a testimony to a past I was not part of. Another life. One I only knew from pictures and Dave and his friends' endless stories. Oh, Dave was so proud of his hair once he had it back! He would wash it every day and took great care over how he styled it – very few people were trusted to touch or trim it. He felt it gave him an identity and became part of his public persona, so losing it all over again twenty-odd years later when he started his treatment for cancer was an incredibly painful cross to bear. The hair given to him after one illness was now being taken away because of another, and he was in pieces when he found clumps on the pillow after his first round of chemotherapy. And then more in the shower.

I decided to spare him that hurt and reached for the razor, convincing him that taking the lead and owning it was the best way forward. We gently shaved it all off and psychologically he felt a lot better making it his decision to get rid of it rather than waiting for cancer and chemo to claim it. It was a small win in his mind and that was enough for me.

* * *

By the time he was 24, Dave had lost both his parents. Jim died in January 1978 after suffering a second stroke and Margaret passed away four years later in a care home. It was left to Dave to clear out the family's council flat, salvaging whatever sentimental items collected over a lifetime he could fit on his Honda 185 Benly.

One of the few precious objects he managed to take with him was a tin dish used by his mum to bake pies in. He kept this tin and treasured it. I wasn't even allowed to touch it! He kept it at the back of the kitchen cupboard and it only ever came out when he was making a pie from one of Margaret's old recipes.

He wasn't left with much at all from his past, which is why it was such a lovely surprise in 2023 during what turned out to be Dave's final months when someone messaged on social media to say they were in possession of one of his very first paintings. It was of a Barrow pub landlady called Joan who used to allow him to sit in a corner of the bar to do his homework as a schoolboy. The painting, now more than 50 years old, made its way to us, a little piece of history.

Dave left his childhood behind as he rode out of Barrow that day in 1982, the bike transporting him to his future. Bikes took him through every experience, connecting the dots, so they always had a huge symbolic significance to him. The end of one chapter and the beginning of another.

By then he was living and working in London, having chosen to remain there after graduating, and those years in the capital were a mixture of studies, odd jobs, dodgy cars, friendships and, best of all for him, an introduction to many new types of food.

Fresh out of uni, he applied for a BBC traineeship in makeup and prosthetics and was the chosen one out of 3,000 applicants! The first male to be taken on the scheme. People are always surprised to learn that long before the Hairy Bikers took off, Dave was a very successful makeup artist across 23 years and his portfolio included top TV series and movies with some of the industry's biggest names.

Specialising in prosthetics and special effects, he was twice nominated for a BAFTA for his work and also trained the next generation of makeup artists, many of whom have gone on to enjoy hugely successful careers themselves. Dave had a bottomless pit of stories about the films and faces that he worked on. Christoper Lambert, Sir Roger Moore, Dennis Hopper, Helen Mirren, Stephanie Beacham, Timothy West, Michael Parkinson, Vanessa Redgrave, Jane Seymour ... the list goes on. And huge series like *The Forsyte Saga* and *Prime Suspect*.

Not so long ago, while I was going through some old pictures with his much-loved makeup-artist friend Suzanna Allaun, we came across a message from Roger Moore, handwritten on a correspondence page from the InterContinental Hotel in Luxembourg.

'My dear David,' it read, 'thank you for taking such good care of my old face! I look forward to repeating the experience.'

Dave once took me to the Luxembourg restaurant he and Sir Roger would dine in together while shooting a movie called *The Enemy*, back in the year 2000. In true Dave form, he remembered every detail of the meals they'd eaten all those years before, and to our amazement, the restaurant still had the same menu. This delighted Dave no end! He even named one of his cars Sir Roger, an old Bentley Continental that had a sat nav set to Mr Moore's gentlemanly tones.

By 1987 he was working as a freelance and had met his first love, Kate, a costume designer, on the set of the Granada TV movie *Breakthrough at Reykjavik*. They married a couple of years later and relocated to the northeast of Scotland, buying an apartment above a small shop in Huntly, Aberdeenshire and setting up an antiques business together. I'm not sure how happy those years were, but they must have loved each other and Dave spoke fondly about the fun he had running the shop, with him taking ad hoc makeup artistry work when he could throughout the year.

However, after being away on a job in Darlington, he returned one weekend to find the shop, flat and his bank account all emptied and Kate gone. Twisting the knife further was the discovery that she'd enlisted the help of Dave's unwitting best friend, Dr Dave Easton, to load the van under the guise of going to an antiques fair. Poor Dr Dave had no idea he was aiding and abetting Kate to clean Dave out and he felt terrible, although of course it wasn't his fault. It would be a source of humour between the two Daves throughout all the years that followed.

Dave never saw Kate again after that and they only spoke once more to agree to an uncontested divorce. From what he told me, she felt unsettled living where they were, but the reality for Dave was now starting his life again from scratch.

Which he did.

* * *

Dave didn't realise it at the time, but 1994 would turn out to be one of the most significant years of his life. He was working on the TV production of Catherine Cookson's *The*

Gambling Man when he immediately hit it off with the series location manager.

This was a certain bloke by the name of Simon King ... and it was the beginning of a beautiful friendship that would take them around the world, bringing the kind of success they could only have dreamed of as boys growing up in Barrow and County Durham. They bonded over their shared love of bikes, food and 'talking bollocks', and over the next few years worked together on a number of productions. Dave was welcomed into Si's family and Si was there when Dave's friendship with script supervisor Glenys – known as Glen – finally turned into romance, thrilled that his best mate was so happy and in love after divorcing Kate.

Dave was besotted with Glen and proposed to her within weeks of them getting together on New Year's Eve 1997, but their happiness proved tragically short-lived. Just days after becoming engaged, Glen fell gravely ill and doctors found a tumour in her stomach. Dave spent three months on a camp bed by her side in hospital as she underwent aggressive treatment and he was with her when she died on 9 May, later describing that moment as if a 'kind of veil had wafted across her'. He was still haunted by this date when I came into his life years later and I became aware of the mournful mood he'd assume on each anniversary of Glen's death.

Losing Glen left him devastated and so he knew exactly what I was feeling 25 years later when he was so desperately poorly himself. He had been in my position. He was watching me caring for him just as he had cared for Glen and I know he wanted to protect me. I've since wondered if that contributed to his unwillingness to talk about dying.

After Glen's death and his own scare with the arachnoid cyst later the same year, Dave felt a need to return to his roots, moving back to Barrow where he bought a house on Roa Island's Piel Street. The makeup-artist work was still keeping him employed, but he'd begun to feel disillusioned with it and was restless for a fresh challenge.

For various reasons, Si was also on the hunt for something new and the two of them started to bounce a few ideas around. They'd been told by people who had seen them cook together that they had something special with their easy, breezy camaraderie and mutual love of good grub ... was there some way of combining food, culture, friendship, humour, travel and bike rides into some sort of pitch for a TV show?

To most it would seem impossible. Improbable at best. And it certainly didn't happen overnight. It was two years after their first conversations that Dave and Si even filmed a pilot on what was a shoestring budget of just £1,200.

But the boys never stopped believing and on the back of that haphazard pilot, which involved a microlight flight, cockles and a lot of laughter, they won a commission from BBC Two to make one episode from Portugal, which aired in January 2005.

It was named *The Hairy Bikers' Cookbook* and viewers were charmed by this pair of down-to-earth, normal blokes.

The rest, you might say, is history.

The Plectrum

23 August 2024

His wallet is still where he left it the morning I took him to hospital for the final time. He knew he wouldn't need it … so it remained on the bedside table and I haven't moved or touched it until now.

I bought it for him a couple of years ago and the black leather has since acquired a patina through age and use. The once-straight edges are now soft and curved, moulded to the shape of Dave's back pocket where he used to carry it. I open it up. His bank cards are neatly aligned in the little compartments although they're all long-cancelled now. There are a few old business cards and two passport-sized photos – one of him with long black hair and one very old picture of me.

While inspecting the inside pockets, something falls on the floor. I pick it up and smile because I recognise it instantly. It's a plectrum, a plastic guitar pick. And a very special one. It carries a drawing of a scorpion on one side and on the other, a name: Rudolf Schenker.

When Dave and I were first courting and talking about our favourite music, I confessed, slightly embarrassed, that I liked Scorpions, a German rock band most famous for their 1990 track 'Wind of Change' about the end of the Cold War and hope for the future. Being Eastern European, the song meant a lot to me and my generation, and I'd been a fan ever since.

Dave immediately bought every one of their albums to get to know them better and it became our thing to listen to their music. He embraced my guilty pleasure and made it ours. Scorpions were our band. Over the years we'd follow them all over Europe – whenever they were touring and we were both free, we'd fly off on a city break to watch them. The first gig we went to was in Hamburg in 2009. We were right in front of the stage in the mosh pit, dancing, jumping and singing along with the many thousands of others, when the lead guitarist Rudy threw a couple of plectrums into the crowd, prompting a mad scramble on the floor.

I didn't get the first one, but I made it my mission to find the second, diving to the ground and then rising triumphantly clutching the precious pick. Dave loved to tell people, 'Lil disappeared for a moment and emerged with one of Rudy's picks, what a moment! That's when I knew she was The One!'

And he carried it in his wallet from that day on.

In the summer of 2017, we got to meet the band in person. We had tickets to see them play at the Roman amphitheatre in Nîmes in the South of France, a town Dave and I loved and where we always stayed at a boutique hotel called Jardins Secrets. It turned out that Scorpions were staying at the same place before the gig, which was such a lovely coincidence, and we couldn't believe our luck when their Scottish tour manager, Bill, recognised Dave and introduced us to the band. Klaus, Rudy, Mathias and the naughty Mikkey Dee, who immediately launched into a long conversation about food with Dave.

On the day of the concert we were given Access All Areas passes, visiting Rudy and Klaus in their dressing rooms backstage and getting a picture with the band in the tunnel leading to the stage. We felt like royalty!

Bill then invited us to see them play in Russia later that year. We had to undergo an interview at the Russian embassy in London to obtain our visas before flying out to Moscow for what would be an amazing few days. We visited Red Square, walked for miles in this frozen city, ate caviar, drank vodka abundantly and admired the beautiful Muscovite metro stations.

Dave fancied eating at the White Rabbit, an upmarket restaurant that he'd heard of where the menu was a bit eccentric. Think swan liver pâté paired with ice-cold vodka. Seriously, the vodka was drunk like water in those places, so we followed the example and, instead of wine, ordered a carafe of vodka. Strangely enough, we didn't get drunk.

Scorpions were huge in Russia, so the concert hall was heaving and we had a great time. Thanks to our AAA passes, we again had access everywhere and when Bill asked us if we'd like tickets to see them in St Petersburg two days later, we jumped at the chance. The boys had filmed in St Petersburg two years earlier while shooting *The Hairy Bikers' Northern Exposure*, so Dave already had a few places in mind for us to visit and a couple of restaurants to try, too.

We bought first-class train tickets from Moscow, which was just as luxurious as flying first class, with slippers for our feet and hot meals served on white linen. Once there, we visited the Hermitage Museum, admired the Fabergé craftsmanship and walked along Nevsky Prospekt, the main boulevard in the city. That was where Dave and Si had ridden an old Russian motorbike with a sidecar and broken down amid busy traffic across multiple lanes. The whole scene was captured on camera and is easily the funniest moment of that series.

Dave wanted to take me to a restaurant they'd filmed in called Cococo. He made a reservation online and we were just being shown to our table when a beautiful lady jumped into Dave's arms and greeted him with an enthusiastic embrace. She was a stunning Russian model as well as the owner of the restaurant and she recognised him from two years ago.

She was beautiful in a vibrant green dress and I was green with jealousy … And Dave? He was like the cat who got the cream. After that, he'd tell everyone how he was loved by Russian models and what a heavenly time he'd had, having shared a passionate kiss with one right in front of his wife!

We went to watch Scorpions again the following day where 'Wind of Change' raised the roof and the audience came together in a passionate wave of hearts and souls.

The only time we saw them play in the UK was when they performed at Mikhail Gorbachev's 80th-birthday gala at the Royal Albert Hall in 2011. Knowing how affected I'd been growing up so close to the Romanian/Russian border and living with the Soviet Union menace, Dave was thoroughly entertained by the idea of taking me and bought us a couple of tickets.

'Just think what your father would say,' he giggled. 'He grew up with the Red Army and now you're going to Gorbachev's birthday party!'

Hosted by Kevin Spacey and Sharon Stone, it was a very glitzy affair where fur-coated guests were adorned with diamonds and the champagne flowed all night. The then England manager Fabio Capello was in attendance and Dave was utterly convinced he'd given me a wave. But the highlight for us was, as ever, the live performance by Scorpions who were revered like gods by Russians.

These were all such good times and I'm trying so hard to keep them alive. Opening the mental drawers that contain treasured memories has been the best medicine in moments of emotional pain after losing Dave and one of the ways I pull myself up from the pit. I can see now that grief is such a complex turmoil of emotions – anger, depression, helplessness, guilt, sorrow, despair – and what helps is separating them all in a conscious way. I think therapy has a big role to play in this. Being part of different groups in my line of work has meant I've always had someone I could easily reach out to and talk with. I realised that one of the battles I was fighting in my head and heart was anger ... There has been a lot of anger and when it comes, the best way to deal with it has been to walk through it.

At times, I've had conversations with myself, analysing the situation and then applying logic. Why am I so angry with myself and with the situation? Was it my inability to do more to stop it? The unfairness of watching this remarkable man lose his light a little bit more every day, until the last breath? Could I have found a cure or some way to postpone the inevitable? Or a tablet he could take to bring it to a halt?

And the answer is no, of course not.

This questioning of and reasoning with myself has helped turn things around in such a way that I understand and accept there was nothing more I could have done. It was out of my hands and the best I could do was to make sure Dave had the care he needed, that his days were as free of pain as they could be and were spent in an environment where he was able to say his goodbyes.

Slowly, slowly, with every question I ask of myself, I can chip away at the anger until I finally start to breathe again. Long walks, time with friends, making plans for stepping forward, it all helps. Having a dog helps too! I don't know where I'd be without Teddy forcing me to get out of the house on days I can barely lift my head off the pillow.

Dave and Me

What an incredible little object this plectrum is. I'm so grateful for the memories it has unveiled today, all such huge moments for us. I'm choosing now to redirect my thoughts to a happier place, which is why I'm back there in that mosh pit in Hamburg. And I'm holding this guitar pick, a symbol of a life lived with intensity and in the spirit of adventure.

Chapter Four

How We Met

Smoother than Brad Pitt on the pull!

When people used to ask me what brought me to the UK, I'd reply, 'A man on his bike.'

That much was true. Dave was biking in my neck of the woods when we first met and we rode bikes around the world throughout our life together. I wasn't looking for him, he just found me. Or maybe we found each other. Perhaps we both offered something the other was hoping to find.

On that fateful day he came into my life in the spring of 2005, I was at work, checking the invoices and payments at the hotel desk. Two large characters walked in, both with long hair and beards, and they filled the small reception area with their large frames. And with their smiles.

Dave and Simon.

They'd been booked to stay somewhere else but hadn't liked it and it had been Si's idea to look for an alternative option. I had no idea who they were – to me they were just two clients seeking accommodation and so I showed them to their rooms, not giving it a second thought apart from being pleased that having them here would give me a chance to practise my English skills.

The only two rooms we had available shared a bathroom, so it was like an apartment which was accessed via a winding staircase. I was wearing a smart business skirt and, as I learned later, Dave took the opportunity to admire my legs as he followed me up.

He told Simon privately afterwards, 'I fancy her!'

I was completely unaware that he'd taken a shine to me – I was just doing my job and wasn't even smiling. Indeed, Simon's response to Dave's admission was to say, 'Mate, she's really scary!' Let me explain. When you work in an environment where you're having to deal with certain customers and often alcohol, you have to be firm and in charge. I therefore always had my business face on at work and so yes, of course I was scary!

It was Dave and Si's first time in Romania and they were starting work on their debut series, *The Hairy Bikers' Cookbook*, which had been commissioned after the Portugal pilot episode had delivered an astonishing 2.7 million viewers for BBC Two. This initial trip was part of a recce and they returned a month later with their crew in tow, booking out the whole hotel this time, to film what became two episodes of the seven-part series.

As it turned out, whatever they'd planned to film in the area had to be cancelled. They'd been relying on sunshine and blue skies and that week the weather had turned nasty, meaning they couldn't take the bikes up on the mountain trails as planned. On the morning they'd been due to start shooting, the team were all gathered in the hotel breakfast room, scratching their heads not knowing what to do. They'd hired a Romanian 'fixer' who travelled with them and helped with local knowledge, but that person wasn't much use.

This is where I stepped in.

Because I'd already known the boys from the first visit, conversation was easier and I suggested some alternative ideas for filming over the next three days, for which they were grateful. Which is how, purely by accident, I became their fixer and interpreter for the whole time they filmed in Maramureş. I knew the places and the people they could work with, I had the local knowledge and contacts, and those few days were different from anything I'd experienced before. We had great fun! It was the first time I'd ridden a motorbike, on the back of Dave's BMW R1200GS as we travelled between locations.

The only other vehicle they travelled in was the very tiny Tico I had access to as a company car. Quite hilariously, Dave and Simon could barely fit their large frames in it and I also clocked them looking very suspiciously at the state of that car with its shattered windscreen and multiple dents. I don't think either believed me when I said, 'It wasn't me!' although I promise that was true. I'm pretty sure they both thought I was a madwoman.

All the locations we filmed at on my recommendation made it into the series, which was quite remarkable – I was thrilled to learn that later. The boys had wanted to film someone cooking a dish called *balmos*, which is traditionally made up in the mountains by the shepherds who herd the sheep. The recipe is simple – sheep's milk and cream boiled in a cauldron with spices and polenta flour.

When it became clear that riding the bikes up in the mountains was out of the question, I found them a Plan B. I took them to a nearby village to see Auntie Ileana, an exceptionally jolly and chatty old lady I knew well. She made them a big cauldron of *balmos*, chatting along while Dave and Si paced around her stove, interested in and liking what they saw. As usual, Ileana was on fire, twittering away merrily and gesturing with her wooden spoon – the boys could only nod and smile because they had no clue what she was talking about.

She didn't wait for any direction, she just took the lead and sat them down at a rickety table, whacked some tin plates in front of them and then sat down herself, shouting at me, 'Hey girl, sit down and quickly grab some food or else these two big bears will eat it all!' Well, I was beside myself. It was so bloody funny. Although obviously I couldn't translate any of that.

Balmos is a savoury dish, served as a main, and after taking a few spoonfuls of what was on their plates, Dave and Si asked what Ileana usually did for dessert. I put the question to her.

'Just a second,' she replied, 'I'll do it.'

She picked up a pot containing caster sugar and plonked two tablespoons onto what was left of the *balmos* on each of the boys' tin plates telling them: 'Eat! This is dessert!' The bemused and bewildered looks on their faces were priceless.

The following day the crew was filming in a village hosting a big feast with a barbecue and locally prepared delicatessen. They'd asked me to find some musicians to generate a bit of an atmosphere and a group of artists arrived shortly afterwards with their instruments. I'd warned the musicians that they weren't supposed to touch the food until filming was over, but it must have fallen on deaf ears. Before I could stop them, they started to demolish the boys' food which had been all beautifully set up for the shot, much to the poor director's exasperation.

Another funny anecdote about Dave's time in Maramureş was something he always told people with great amusement. While searching for a cashpoint in the town, he'd been accosted by the local 'character' (every town has one) who, at the time, was holding a plastic bag full of cabbages.

Sussing that Dave was a foreigner, he said: 'Hello, I'm Antonio Banderas, who are you?' Dave quipped back, 'Hello Antonio, I'm Phil Collins.'

This guy had not been expecting a comeback like that and in his shock, he became aggressive, shouting, 'Fuck you, Phil Collins!' and hitting Dave with the bag of cabbages.

It all ended up a pantomime-style fight, to the delight of the large crowd who had gathered to watch the whole ridiculous scene unfold. How I wish I could have been there to witness it too!

I was very sad as they reached the end of filming and the crew packed up their gear to head off on their next journey. I'd had a great time with them all and had enjoyed my rides as pillion on Dave's bike very much. I'd also loved learning about how a piece of TV was produced and watching Dave and Si and the dynamic between them. The conversation in front of the camera was completely unscripted, it just flowed so naturally and I found it quite mesmerising. I'd never met two people as interested in our culture, history and, my goodness, the *food* as they'd been.

After they left, I stayed in touch with Belinda, who was the production manager, and we exchanged a few courtesy emails. She must have passed on my address because one day I had a lovely surprise when I received a short email from Dave thanking me for being so kind and helping them out. I replied politely – after all, it was my job to keep in touch with clients and make sure they were happy with the service they'd received.

It just developed from there.

His emails started to arrive from different parts of the world, wherever the filming was taking them. I was reading about the people of Turkey, the spices of India, the colours of Mexico and the penguins of Patagonia. All these wonderful places, described so beautifully by Dave and capturing my imagination.

Dear Lili,

Just a quick note from Vietnam. We have been here for two weeks now doing research, and it is going very well.

It's a difficult country to crack as the people are very reserved, but the food is amazing. It's much finer than Chinese food and not so spicy as Thai.

We got up at dawn today to go to a Tai Chi class underneath Lenin's statue in the middle of town. What a sight the size of us two in the middle of all the tiny Vietnamese folk doing their early morning exercises.

I like Hanoi, but Saigon is very, very busy and humid.

I hope all is well and OK in Romania. Have you received a DVD yet? If not, mail me and I will sort it out for you.

Lots of love from the Far East,
David

I'd always dreamed of travelling and now I was seeing the world through his eyes because he was such a good story-teller. The more he wrote, the more he revealed about himself, and although Dave's reality was so different to mine and the whole world was squashed between us, I understood that he was a truly special person, full of warmth, wisdom and spark.

He was a charming, witty and joyous writer and I found myself looking forward to his messages, to the point where they became very important for me. His emails brought magic into my life.

And then on 28 December 2005 (which just happened to be my 39th birthday), he called me on my mobile. He hadn't known it was my birthday, it was a complete coincidence, but it felt quite nice to get a phone call from abroad on that day. We chatted for a short while – he told me he was going to spend New Year's Eve in Dublin and I said I'd be working as the hotel was playing host to a big party. It was a warm, short but sweet phone call and would be the first of many.

Over the next few months, we spoke on the phone regularly, developing a great deal of affection for each other, and so when he invited me to visit him at his home in Barrow-in-Furness in March 2006, I was delighted to accept. It was the first time I'd ever been abroad, the first time I'd even been on a plane.

Because Romania was not in the EU back then, I had to go to the embassy for a day of interviews in order to get a visa. I prepared a huge file detailing my financial and employment status and the situation with my kids, and Dave had to send me letters from the BBC along with his bank statements to qualify as my 'sponsor' for the visit. It was still just a friendship between us; I thought it would be a nice holiday and a chance to meet up again with everyone from the show.

He greeted me at Manchester Airport with a big Dave hug (Dave always had a hug for everyone) and drove me to his home in Barrow. It was about midnight when we got to his house and, knowing I was hungry, he offered to make me a sandwich. Dave's kitchen was crammed with all sorts of gadgets, utensils, plates, pots and stacks of spice jars. I'd never been cooked for by a man and now here was Dave, making the most perfect sandwich imaginable, just for me. I don't remember what ingredients he used to create such loveliness, but my god, it tasted divine. He always had the skill to take simple ingredients found in any fridge and turn them into something sophisticated and fulfilling.

Looking back, I think that sandwich might have sealed the deal for me. Watching him pour his heart and soul into it, taking such care to perfect it … well, he opened a new world to me – his world – of tastes, smells and textures. Food for me had only ever been about survival and necessity, but Dave showed me that it could be art. And love.

He served love on a plate!

During my fortnight in the UK, we went to London, over to Newcastle to meet Si and his wife, Jane, and up to Scotland to visit Dave's best friend, Dr Dave, and his family in Aberdeenshire. It all felt so easy and he made me feel safe.

Dave was the perfect gentleman and a lovely person to talk to and travel with. He had a Mercedes-Benz S-Class he'd named Maria after one of the folk musicians we'd filmed with in Romania. This Maria lady had a very pitchy voice and as she'd sung, she'd waved her hands about all fluttery, in a similar movement to the windscreen wipers on Dave's Merc. That made me laugh.

It was around the time the boys' debut book was coming out and this was a massive milestone for Dave, particularly because the Barrow branch of Waterstones had displayed a big promotional poster of him and Si. We were out for a stroll when he saw it in the window and he was so happy! I took a photo of him next to it, giving it the thumbs-up.

I knew we were developing strong feelings for each other, but I warned him not to fall in love with me. There were too many obstacles stacked against us: we were from different worlds and I had two children back home to think of – by this time Sergiu was 16 and Iza 10. I kept my guard up and treated what we had as a friendship for quite a long time. For me at least, it was a slow-burn which grew into something beautiful and an emotional stability, which was a feeling I'd not experienced before.

Dave exuded so much charm and happiness that I gradually realised how much had been lacking in my life. Tales of the experiences he had filming and the people he'd met on those journeys spoke so much about him as a person – I had never known anyone like him, with so much vivacity, so much love to give and such a generous heart. His decisions and actions were never self-centred or self-indulgent, he was always respectful of others, consistent and safe to be around. It was impossible not to like Dave Myers! And, so it turned out for me, impossible not to fall in love with him either.

Despite my warnings, both of us were helpless to it.

Dave brought adventure and spontaneity into my life for the first time. In May 2006 we went to Si's brother's wedding in Italy, Dave riding from England, me flying in from Romania and meeting him in Pisa, where I joined him on the bike to travel onwards to Figline Valdarno. My return flight from Florence three days later was cancelled due to an Air Italia strike but I found one for the following day from Milan. So, we got back on the bike and rode there from Florence.

'This is a stolen day for us,' said Dave. He went online and, on a whim, booked the poshest hotel in Milan he could find. It was called Villa San Carlo Borromeo and was where the Pope traditionally stayed while visiting the city.

'I can't afford it,' he said, 'but we're going to have it.'

It was such a lot of money for one night and we looked so out of place at this exquisite hotel, with its beautiful gardens and Renaissance paintings, where even the bellboys wore Armani suits. My bag was tied with rope, I was in sloppy clothes having been expecting to fly, and we were both dishevelled and coated in dust from the road. We stifled giggles as the staff lugged our old bags onto the ornate trolley to be taken to our room.

We had dinner in the restaurant that night, and it was exceptional. What a treat and such an unexpected one. We loved it so much, this stolen day, that we returned to the same hotel the following year for Dave's 50th, this time taking Dr Dave, his wife and two friends from Barrow.

By the late spring of 2006 we were speaking on the phone at least twice a day and Dave would be sure to call me even if it was only for a minute or two. I so looked forward to hearing his voice, it was the best part of my day and so when he failed to make contact for 48 hours, I became worried. Had I done something wrong? Or had something bad happened to him? I eventually got a call from Dr Dave to tell me that Dave had been airlifted to hospital after a serious motorbike accident.

The pair of them had gone to the Isle of Man Tourist Trophy, a two-week annual motorcycle event for bike enthusiasts known to be one of the most dangerous racing events in the world. It used to feature an informal, death-defying free-for-all called Mad Sunday where spectators could tear around the town and mountainous course in any vehicle at any speed. Crazy.

There were multiple casualties every year and this time Dave was one of them following a collision with a lorry on a bend known ominously as Devil's Elbow, which had sent him and his bike flying. Dr Dave, who had been riding just behind, witnessed the whole thing which must have been horrific for him. The only part of Dave's Benelli Tornado Italian superbike left in one piece was a mirror.

'I don't want you to be worried, Lil,' said Dr Dave on the phone. 'He's alive, he's OK.' He'd somehow escaped with just a broken shoulder, a broken wrist and some internal bleeding, and was so lucky to have survived. I wanted to fly out immediately; I felt I should be there and that he needed me – he had his right shoulder and left wrist in splints and was unable to do anything for himself.

But Si moved in for a few days and took care of him, even washing him in the shower while Dave jokingly sang '*Je t'aime … moi non plus*', the steamy track by Serge Gainsbourg and Jane Birkin.

'Look, if anything moves *down there*,' warned Si, 'I'm out of here!'

I think the strength of my feelings – the worry that he was hurt, the relief that he was OK and then my instinctive need to come over to be with him – were a clear sign to me that this relationship was intensifying.

Another wonderful trip away came just before Christmas in 2006 when I joined Dave for the weekend in Brussels where he and Si were filming for their third series, *The Hairy Bikers Ride Again*. Beneath gentle snowflakes, we ate chocolate truffles and drank champagne while watching passers-by and admiring the splendid architecture of the buildings surrounding the square. The Grand-Place is quite rightly considered one of the most beautiful places in the world. If you've ever been there during the festive season, you'll know that they have the most stunning tree right in the middle of the market and when we were there, visitors could take a little tin-foil star and write a wish on it to hang on one of the branches which were all lit up in blue. My wish was that Dave and I would one day return here together. I don't know what Dave wrote on his and I won't ever know now ... but I like to think that he wished for the same.

Some people say that there is no perfect match, we just make it perfect by doing the right thing. And there is truth in all of this: you make the choice to make a change. Dave and I had the courage to do just that. My relocation to the UK the following year was a huge decision for us – as a mother, my children, who were 17 and 11 at that point, had always been my priority and this would mean putting myself first and altering their whole futures in the process. But Dave and I both felt that this was worth investing in. He made me feel adored in so many ways, from describing what he felt when he first saw me, to telling me how his eyes had welled with tears when I first sewed a loose button on his favourite shirt.

I never felt anything other than loved and valued.

He accepted me completely – my qualities and my imperfections – and in his wise and gentle way he made me understand that I didn't need to be on guard all the time, that it was OK to relax and be myself. He helped me to love fully and to allow myself to be loved. We were two people making their way through life hand in hand, in the purest and most authentic way possible.

There was only one next logical step. I started to make plans to move to Barrow.

The Book

1 September 2024

It's gloomy and wet outside and there's very little light coming in through the window here in the study. As much as I'd like to feel enthusiastic about the various jobs that need my attention, the weather reflects my mood. Grief comes in waves and in different shapes. One day it's pure fatigue, on others it's heavy sadness or nostalgia. That part of it is unpredictable.

What I do know is that it's here to stay so I'd better make friends with it and accept that it is now part of me forever. You can't sweep grief under the carpet or kick it down the road. It will only fester and corrode and then unleash itself without warning. There is a vast body of literature on the subject of grief and loss and, in my journey to find my peace, I've read a great deal of books and listened to many experts talking about this. I learned about the five stages of grief identified by Elisabeth Kübler-Ross in *On Death and Dying* – denial, anger, bargaining, depression and acceptance. David Kessler added a sixth stage (finding meaning) in *Finding*

Meaning: The Sixth Stage of Grief. In his short manuscript *A Grief Observed*, C.S. Lewis questioned identity, faith and the meaning of life after losing his wife, while Julia Samuel wrote about how people process grief and navigate life's emotional challenges in *Grief Work: Stories of Life, Death and Surviving.*

All have offered me invaluable insights as to how one might face loss, but when you're in the depths of it yourself, you realise there's no set pattern, no exact science. Grief doesn't follow a perfect timeline and we don't move through bereavement in anything like an orderly fashion. Nor should we try to.

I'm doing my best ... that's what I keep telling myself and everyone else. Take it easy, one step at a time. There's a mountain of things to be sorted, though. Not just mentally in the compartments of my mind, but practically in the house too, dealing with the aftermath of Dave's passing. Solicitors, probate, banks, mortgage lenders, insurance companies, the DVLA and utilities providers – all this paperwork is another layer of pressure thrown on top of the grief.

In the modern world there are also passwords, computers, phones and increasingly more to resolve. It's the correspondence coming through the door saying: 'Dear Mrs Myers, we are so sorry for your loss, but ...' Or, 'In the wake of your husband passing, you need to send us these documents ...' It's awful opening such a letter, so devoid of feelings and making the situation so brutally real. Like a transaction.

It's as if I must untangle everything, wipe the slate clean and neatly close down his life. I have to make decisions I'm not ready for about his car and his motorbikes. And what to do with the medicine, pills and potions that are scattered everywhere, reminders of pain and illness and of false hopes that they could perform a miracle and bring back the good days.

I need something to divert my attention from all this commotion in my head and help me reconnect with Dave in some way that isn't via pain. I want to feel the happiness we once experienced … which brings me to his bookcase. I bought this IKEA unit for him as a Christmas present a few years back and built it on my own. At the time we were having some work done in the house and I remember the tradesmen were laughing at me unpacking the screwdrivers and the numerous parts I had to put together and they offered to help.

'No, no, I'm going to do it myself for my husband, thank you!' I replied.

Dave was awfully pleased with the gift and we used it to display all the trophies and awards he won with Si, as well as the many he received on his own. It's a mighty impressive collection and he loved showing it to visitors. On the top shelf there are no fewer than five Fortnum & Mason Personality of the Year awards – Dave was hugely appreciative of these because they were voted for by the public. An added bonus was the fact that the F&M parties were glamorous and fun to attend and the award would be followed by the arrival of a luxury hamper filled with delicious treats.

I have a stack of those woven baskets bearing the F&M logo in the orangery.

There's a TV Choice trophy for Best Food Show (for *Bakeation*) from 2012, various book of the year awards for *The Hairy Dieters*, two *Through the Keyhole* trophies, and a silver carriage clock from our 2013 appearance on *All Star Mr and Mrs*. Dave used to say that we were the worst couple they'd ever had on the show because every one of our answers about each other was wrong! I'd struggled to understand the convoluted questions that host Phillip Schofield was asking me and hadn't been able to reply in time, so it was all quite disastrous. Still, we came away with that bedazzled clock for our troubles and I have to say that, more than ten years on, it still keeps perfect time.

The one Dave was proudest of was the blue crystal *Celebrity Mastermind* trophy from 2008. Despite everyone warning him not to do it and his terror that the sound of the dramatic music and the intensity of the spotlight would combine to wipe his mind blank, Dave signed up to the show. I was in the studio audience and my heart sank when host John Humphrys' first words to him were, 'So, you're two fat, hairy blokes who like riding motorbikes, and somebody bought that as a TV show?' I felt sure the sneeriness would throw him off and he would lose focus, but Dave always had a smart answer on the tip of his tongue and he replied, 'Well, John, as well as riding bikes, we like cooking, travelling and having a chat, and I hope we're encouraging other people to give it a go, too!'

Oh, the triumphant look on his face when he won and was handed that gong! His plan, if there was ever a *Mastermind of the Mastermind* follow-up show, was to nominate *SpongeBob SquarePants* as his specialist subject.

There are also awards that I've picked up on his behalf when he was no longer strong enough to do it himself and more since he passed such as the Cumbria Personality of the Year 2024. Those moments are always full of mixed emotions for me. Pride, gratitude, sadness.

This bookcase is home to decades of work, knowledge, courage and determination. I only wish he'd been able to add all the accolades he won in his life as a makeup artist before I met him. He kept pictures of the faces and characters he'd worked on, but there are no awards that I can proudly place alongside everything else.

The lower shelves of the bookcase house a pristine copy of every book the boys wrote across their Hairy Bikers career which I bought online to display. All of them in order. And there are a lot of them! I don't think it's a coincidence that I feel drawn to one in particular today. *Blood, Sweat and Tyres* is the autobiographical story of the boys' lives and when it came out in 2015, I must admit I didn't read it. While Dave was writing it, he'd read passages out to me – these were stories I'd heard many times before because we'd always talked about his past and the impact his childhood had on his life.

'You want to know anything about me, read my book!' he used to joke.

'I'm not going to read a book where I only have half a page and Karen from *Strictly Come Dancing* has seven!' I'd tease him in reply.

Well, now is the time to read it because I want to try to find Dave again in a different way. His words, his humour, whatever it was that he managed to capture within the pages of this book – I'm looking for something I didn't know about him. Or maybe something I did know but have forgotten … a reconnection. I'm enthralled from the very first page. There's an ease with which Dave communicates, simple stories flowing in a way that creates atmosphere and colour, and I find his vocabulary and tone so very familiar. I can remember him telling me some of the stories in the same words and with the same verve and wit.

I can picture his lips, stopping to take a breath every now and again, pausing for comic effect, stroking his moustache and beard while talking. I can see the twinkle in his eyes and I can feel the fun he'd weave into every story. His face would light up when he spoke about his parents or told a tale from his travels, a smile always waiting in the corners of his mouth, ready to become a hearty laugh when he got to the punchline.

Large parts of Dave's life were complex and challenging, but he recounts all this in such an uncomplicated way and knowing I was part of the process as he wrote this book … well, it connects us. I remember him working on it when we were on holiday in France over the spring of 2014, writing during the day and in the evening cooking beautiful meals, washed down with a glass of Condrieu. He was in good health and full of the Dave Myers vibrance. He was happy, *we* were happy. We were safe.

Then it hits me. That's what I'm looking for!

It's the feeling of safety I had when Dave was strong and full of energy. Reading his words is bringing me the comfort of familiarity I've been craving. That's what I've been missing. I have found safety in Dave's words and they are my anchors to happier times. The future is so uncertain and scary and I can't map it out right now, but maybe finding these connections to the past will somehow light the way. I carry on reading. I read the whole book.

And I remind myself there's no need to rush to resolve everything right now. Some things can wait. One step at a time!

Chapter Five

Making the Move

The water jumps around in the pan like a Morris dancer with worms!

I still get goosebumps thinking back to the time I upped sticks and moved to the UK. It wasn't easy, nor was it without pain, leaving everything behind. The kids had – and have always maintained – a close relationship with their father and I never wanted to do anything to come between that.

Iza was just 11 and I was taking her away from everything familiar and bringing her to a new town in a new country where she didn't speak the language. This was my decision, not hers, and it would have huge consequences for both of our lives.

Complicating that decision further was the fact that Sergiu was just about to take his Baccalaureate exams in Romania and would have to be left behind while he completed his education. He did join us in the UK the following year, but as a mother my heart was split in two heading to Barrow without him.

I was riddled with guilt and taking a huge leap of faith, not least because Dave's line of work was not your average nine-to-five and would mean he was often away. And yet somehow, I found the courage to make that life-changing move and dive into the unknown without looking back. I'm not sure if I could ever trust one person again as much as I did Dave in that moment, two years after we'd first met. Two years of long-distance emails, phone calls and falling in love.

Dave took on the responsibility of making things work for all of us. He was always so good at doing the right thing, at finding solutions to make everybody happy and engineering the best and brightest situation out of something knotty and complicated. He was a visionary, able to predict how things would evolve and it was such a beautiful thing to trust his judgement implicitly and know everything would turn out right.

So, on 3 September 2007, Iza and I packed our lives into two large suitcases, said our tearful farewells and headed to the airport. The big move didn't get off to the most auspicious of starts. Due to circumstances outside of our control, we missed our connecting flight from Heathrow to Manchester, delaying our arrival by more than two hours. And although we eventually landed safely, unfortunately our luggage did not – that was still sitting on the tarmac in London. What a start to my new life in the UK! After a stressful journey, the news about our bags pushed me to the brink and I called

Dave who was waiting patiently for us on the other side of arrivals, a bunch of flowers in his hand.

'Darling,' I said, my voice quivering, 'we are here but I have one little girl, one handbag, no money and nothing to my name. Not even a suitcase. If you don't want us, tell me and we'll go back to where we came from right now.'

I was tired, hungry, on the verge of tears and fully prepared to turn back. But my man was my rock, in that moment and for all the years to come.

'Oh, darling, don't be daft,' he said gently. 'I'm not going anywhere; I'm right here waiting for both of you.'

He had an innate ability to calm, always managing to find the right words. After filling in a load of lost-luggage forms, we made our way to the exit where Dave greeted us with that lovely big grin of his. My heart leapt when I saw him and I just knew everything was going to be OK as he drove us to Barrow-in-Furness in Maria the Mercedes, characteristically full of beans and chatting at nineteen to the dozen!

Dave's home – which was now our home too – was on Roa Island, off the coast of Barrow. There were only about 20 houses on the island, a café, a guesthouse and a lifeboat station. To me, the house was huge, with its two reception rooms, lounge and kitchen on the ground floor and three large bedrooms plus a big family bathroom complete with free-standing bathtub on the second.

It was late by the time we arrived and our new reality kicked in quickly. Iza didn't understand English and Dave couldn't speak Romanian, so I had to interpret whatever they were saying. Picture this. In his excited kid-in-a-toy-shop way, Dave was showing us around the house and was practically jumping for joy as he opened the door to what was now Iza's bedroom. Since I'd last visited, he'd transformed it into a pink paradise – there was a new pink desk, pink chair, pink bicycle ... pink everything.

My daughter asked me in Romanian, 'What's this? I hate pink!'

'What did she say?' asked Dave expectantly.

'That she loves it!' I lied, not having the heart to spoil his moment.

I must admit though, Iza made her feelings perfectly clear by her face. Things didn't get much better in the kitchen, where Dave set the table and prepared us each one of his elaborate sandwiches which Iza point blank refused to eat.

'I just want bread and butter,' she declared, disregarding all the good food on the table. She would only eat bread and butter for the first few weeks, to Dave's confusion and dismay, but food was different and unfamiliar here and Iza was looking for ways of feeling closer to our old life. Bless her. My girl really was in at the deep end. She was starting her new school in just a few days' time, so she had an awful lot to get her head around.

Also, Dave then had to leave to go away with work for a whole week. Ouch. Not exactly great timing, but he and Si were in the middle of filming their third series, *Hairy Bikers*

Dave and Me

Ride Again, and were also due to attend a charity ball where they were the guests of honour. I'd always known his schedule was going to be full on, but it was a baptism of fire all the same. He'd bought me a Honda Civic runaround to ferry Iza to and from school, but I'd never driven a right-handed car before on the other side of the road, let alone in a town I didn't know.

I had to find my way to the school on that first day using a physical map on the dashboard because this was before cars came equipped with sat navs. Not only did I make it to the school and deliver Iza on time, I also managed to fill up the car with fuel AND then pop to the local Tesco. I was so proud of myself! I felt for Iza as she walked through the school gates for the first time, the nerves swirling around my chest. Although we didn't have much money back then, Dave was determined to give her the best start and had cobbled together the funds to put her into private school.

On that first Monday morning, she announced that she hated the uniform – the striped blazer and pleated skirt – although she went on to wear it with pride for the next seven years. Everything was peculiar to her and I know the kids at school looked at her with curiosity because she was different.

While Dave was away that week, I tried to keep her spirits up and, as a treat, took her out to eat. I didn't know many places in town and so we ended up having a meal at the café in Morrisons where I was also doing a bit of shopping. Well, Dave was howling on the phone when I told him.

'There are so many nice restaurants and you only found Morrisons?!' he chuckled.

It had made sense to me to eat there because it was convenient and cheap, but there were other things at play here. I'd never had experiences like this, being able to go where I wanted, when I wanted, have the things I wanted and not really worry about the cost. In terms of money, my only point of reference was still the one I'd grown up with and if I was paying ten pounds for a meal in the UK, I couldn't stop myself from calculating how much that would be in Romanian Leu. It was scary to spend that much on myself and it took a long time to get over the scarcity mindset and my habit of comparing values in the two currencies.

In the beginning, whatever money we had in the bank was used towards school fees, the mortgage and day-to-day living. To me though, it was a fortune and it meant stability, safety, peace of mind. My man was creative and hardworking – his efforts were making us comfortable; we had a nice home, a car and endless love for each other. I knew I could trust him with my life and my kids' lives, and he knew he'd come home to my loving embrace. I had his back and he had my safety.

I was building him a home, he was building us security.

It was going to take time to acclimatise, though. A couple of weeks after we arrived, I picked Iza up from school and she was a bit upset.

'What's the matter?' I asked her. 'Tell me why you're sad.'

'Some of the boys have been laughing at me because I can't speak their language,' she replied.

'Would you like me to go and speak to your teachers about it?'

She was adamant that I shouldn't. She'd manage it herself.

And, with the help of an English tutor, she picked everything up super quickly. About six months after she started, we received a letter from the school saying that she no longer needed extra help.

'What do the boys at school say now, Iza?' I asked her. 'Are they still laughing?'

She smiled.

'As if they'd dare,' came the steely reply.

That's when I knew that whatever happened, my feisty little girl was going to do just fine. When she turned 12 in the June after we arrived, she asked if she could take a few friends to the cinema. 'A few' meant 24! While the kids were at the movies, Dave prepared food at home and when the parents came to collect their children, they all stayed to eat as well. And when I say stayed … it was about midnight before everyone left and *that* was only when the grandparents had arrived to pick them up! What a fantastic indication of how far we'd all come.

* * *

Over that first year in the UK, we gradually found our feet and managed to adapt to this new way of living. On days between filming, Dave helped us in every step of the process, introducing me to our neighbours and to his friendship group. He often told the story of him taking me for a Chinese for the first time in my life. It was at the Diamond restaurant on Dalton Road and was run by Jim and Lily, who became good friends of ours. I'd never tasted a prawn before and, oh my word, Dave was utterly bemused as I popped one into my mouth, watching the expression on my face change from surprise to delight! There were so many of these moments – these foodie firsts – and Dave thoroughly enjoyed witnessing my reactions to various taste buds being ignited.

He took me to the Multicultural Community Centre in town, which is where I made so many beautiful friends, people who had moved to Barrow from all different parts of the world. Unlike my hometown where, apart from a smattering of Hungarian and Ukrainian, you never heard any other language or experienced other cultures, Barrow had an awful lot to offer. Thanks to that community centre, I became part of a brilliant group of women – we must have been from about 40 different countries between us and everyone brought something wonderful with them.

I come from a big family, one which always had a lot of social interaction, so I needed to put something in place for me and Iza; a network for us so we weren't completely alone when Dave was away. Something that would give me and my girl structure, a community that was there just for us. I got involved with organising all sorts of events – dancing, food, family days – and it made my heart full to be part of such a friendly and proactive group. I also later trained as an interpreter and started working for Cumbria County Council which in turn led to me becoming involved with the police and child protection.

For all the differences, in a lot of ways Barrow was similar to the town I grew up in, especially the people who I found genuine, smiley and warm. I made friends easily and was charmed by the locals with their kindness and chatty natures. Although everything was new to me, it felt safe.

I remember the night Dave took me into town to the Ormsgill Inn for my first pint in a British pub. There were four or five men in their seventies, not many teeth between them, playing cards and they invited me to join in. Dave came back from the bar to find me having a good laugh with these jolly souls.

'Ah, you've conquered it already,' he smiled. 'Look at you with your admirers!'

It really wasn't long before I felt at home, although there were a couple of things I needed time to get used to. The first was the Cumbrian accent, which took me a good few weeks to tune into – to me it sounded like a squashed version of English. We found it funny when we realised that in our family, English was spoken with four different nuances – mine with an Eastern European accent, Iza with a strong Cumbrian influence (I guess hers was the closest to Dave's), while Sergiu, who went to study computer science in Aberdeen, developed a decidedly Scottish twang.

The other thing I struggled with was the weather. When we first moved to Roa Island, I was excited to be living just a few metres from the sea and in my head I was planning days of bathing and basking in the sun. Haha! Not once, in almost four years of living on Roa, was I able to do that. I quickly realised that the angry Irish Sea and the ever-cloudy sky were always going to laugh in the face of my naive plans.

We had a very small courtyard at the back of the house and in the first year of living there I raised a bed in a corner, trying to grow some tomatoes and onions just as I'd done in Romania. But here, nothing ever grew to maturity; it was all killed by the salt, rain and lack of sun. Yes, weather was a tricky thing indeed.

* * *

Sharing my life with Dave also meant sharing my home with bikes. 'Owning motorcycles is a bit like murder,' he used to say, 'it gets easier after the first few!'

There was the BMW R 1200 GS, the Aprilia Falco 1000cc, our beloved Moto Guzzi California … at one point I think there were ten bikes in our garage. And one in the kitchen. That red MV Agusta was an object of art for Dave and it sat there on a support system in the kitchen. The only time he ever rode it was to bring it home from the place he bought it from in Skipton. It was too beautiful to ride, but every time we had guests for dinner and Dave had a glass of wine too many, he'd rev the engine and the fumes killed all my lovely plants.

Dave and Me

One night he got a little bit *too* merry and ended up impulsively selling it to our friend Mark. The conversation went a little something like this:

Dave: 'I love you, mate!'

Mark: 'I love you, too! And I love your bike!'

Dave: 'Do you want it?'

Sold.

Boy, did he regret it in the morning. But Dave was always a man of his word; when he promised something, he had to deliver and so the Agusta was duly wheeled out of our kitchen and taken to its new home. I've got to admit, I secretly missed that bike too. I'd grown rather fond of it and by that time my plants were all dead anyway, so I had nothing left to lose!

I fell in love with biking very early on in my relationship with Dave. It was the freedom and thrill of it all, never better epitomised than on our annual group trips with the Sons of Royalty who organise charity bike rides in aid of Childline. They are epic journeys which we came to love very much and which gifted us many special friends over the years.

I remember one year crossing the Rockies at about two in the afternoon when we all stopped by the road to watch the solar eclipse. That moment, experienced as a collective, was something else. When you're in a group like that, there is such a special kind of unity where you trust each other with your lives. It's such a great feeling knowing you are part of this community and that this is your tribe – friendship, biking and music: what's not to love?

At home, whenever he had time, Dave would spend hours tinkering with his bikes, polishing them until they gleamed. 'Come on, Lil,' he'd say. 'Grab your helmet and let's go!' And off we'd go, with no destination in mind, just us and the open road. We'd often end up at the Lakes for lunch or enjoying the market in Lancaster.

For the boys' Christmas special in 2008, Dave had a custom-built chopper made called the Myers Superior. This thing was enormous and completely impractical, but Dave was in love. The noise it made could wake the dead! If he ever set off riding it at the crack of dawn, he'd have the entire population of Roa Island up with a single rev of the engine.

Ah, the days when Dave was home were like magic.

He was a man of routine, getting up each morning somewhere between seven and half past and pondering the same question, 'What are we eating today?' That was his first concern. And he didn't just mean for breakfast, he meant for the entire day and he'd begin planning every meal in his head, making a mental list of what ingredients were needed. Dave loved a list. He had them everywhere – paper notes in his pockets and on his desk or typed and stored in his phone.

He'd merrily jump out of bed and I'd watch him go about his morning rituals, darting from one side of the room to the other, drying his hair after showering, grooming his beard and waxing his moustache, carefully lifting up the tips on each side and curling them around his finger. Then he'd choose his socks and a handkerchief from the selection he kept in the top drawer and scoop up the coins that had fallen out of his trousers onto the floor the night before. You'd always hear Dave before you saw him, jangling with all the change he carried in his pockets.

He'd have a copious breakfast and, after dropping Iza at school, we'd go shopping for anything he needed to cook with that day. It didn't matter if we had meat in the freezer, it had to be bought fresh and it had to be the best. Even bacon sarnies had to be made with 'proper' bacon from the butchers, not bought in a packet at the supermarket.

When we returned, Dave would sit himself down at his antique dark-wood Biedermeier desk to write a magazine-commissioned article or to work on some recipes for the boys' latest cookbook. Every Hairy Bikers' book was written at that desk, a surviving piece from the days when Dave traded antiques and which followed us to every house we lived in. All the drawers were stuffed with cards, paperwork and old tapes and it also had secret compartments with tiny ivory knobs and a writing surface you could put up or down.

'What time would you like your dinner?' he'd ask at about 4pm each day.

'About seven, darling,' I'd reply.

'No problem!'

As if. Dinner was rarely served before eight following Dave's tireless efforts to create something different and amazing. I can honestly say in all our time together, I never ate the same dinner twice. He was so innovative, so curious about new combinations and that meant our food coming to us much later than planned, but way more awesome than expected.

It would often take two hours to clean the kitchen after he'd cooked. Dave somehow managed to use every pot and pan, every measuring spoon and set of scales, and there would be remnants of the meal splashed up the walls and even on the ceiling. The price to pay for eating such beautiful food every evening! At times I tried to clean in between his cooking so that the Mount Everest stack of washing up was easier at the other end, but Dave never flinched at the mess and chaos. All that mattered to him was what was on the plate, that was the art.

'My darling,' he would say, 'I am an artist, not a cleaner! At work that is someone else's job, not mine.'

He put so much thought into creating a dish and all his ingredients were treated with the utmost respect. It was always different, always inventive, always *outstanding*. If it was any less than that, it would invariably end up in the bin.

Meal preparation would usually begin with a search online for a recipe for whatever he wanted to make. He'd print that off and then find alternative versions in three or four different books, making notes of the variations, whether that was the spices used, ingredient quantities or cooking times. He'd have all these books open on the cooking surface while he scurried about the kitchen, experimenting, making notes, tasting, building.

'That needs a little more heat – hang on, I'm just going to try a smidge of this, now a touch of that in here ...' And so, the final creation wouldn't be any single one of the recipes he'd looked at, but a combination of all the best bits of several different versions of the same dish and that was how he did it.

If he really liked the result, he would say, 'That's good enough for our next book.' I liked to sit there with a glass of wine, watching him put together these sublime meals. 'Let me make you something nice while you wait, darling,' he'd say. 'Just to put you in the mood.' And he'd prepare me a little sandwich or a petit four with salmon and capers.

Everything was an experience with Dave and when we at last sat down for dinner, he wanted to hear that I enjoyed whatever it was he'd created. 'Tell me that you love it,' he'd say hopefully. 'Please!' He wanted me to be blown away from the very first mouthful and he'd look at me intently, waiting to see my reaction. 'How does it taste? How's the spice balance? Is it too salty? Too peppery? Does it need a little bit more heat? Could it do with some extra pepper? Perhaps some cardamom?' You could say I was his personal food critic because he pushed me to be and he always valued my feedback, even on the rare occasions when it wasn't quite what he wanted to hear.

The carnage in the kitchen was another level entirely when Dave and Si were both there, putting their heads together and perfecting the latest recipes. Those were the best of days, not just for the culinary creations I had the privilege of sampling first, but also for the atmosphere, the naughty jokes and infectious laughter.

They also made the neighbours happy because after writing, cooking, tasting, adjusting and cooking again, I'd be tasked with distributing everything we couldn't eat ourselves to the people who lived close by. We were *very* popular, as I'm sure you can imagine!

* * *

Soon after moving in, Dave took me to his friend and solicitor Paul to write a will, officially making me part of his life. When picking Iza up from school later that day, he tried to explain to her what a will was for and, hilariously, she replied in the few English words she'd picked up.

'So, you die, me rich? Watch your step!'

It was a lovely moment between them, the first sparkle of wit from Iza in English and a bit of a breakthrough for their relationship. Initially, she was naturally very protective of me and if we were out anywhere as a family, she would sit in between Dave and me, pushing us apart. She also wanted me to sleep with her in her bed, which I did – anything to help her feel more settled.

It was Dave who came up with the genius idea of finding a little friend for Iza. A furry one. They both searched online and found a West Highland terrier breeder near Ipswich who just so happened to have a new litter. Within days we set off to have a look at the pups and as soon as we walked through the door, this gorgeous four-week-old bundle of fun ran towards Iza. It was love at first sight. A few weeks later, when we brought Snowy (as Iza had named him) home for the first time, I was finally allowed to share a bed with Dave. Snowy was a gorgeous pet and gave us many years of love.

Once Iza was able to understand the language and got to know Dave, the two of them became the best of friends. They had a ball. Every morning he would make her a dippy egg and soldiers – that was her favourite – and they'd sit on the sofa together watching *SpongeBob SquarePants*. They had the same sense of humour, the same childish natures, and Iza matured into an intelligent and quick-witted young lady. More so than I ever was. Dave was her playmate and I adored watching them together, playing games of Monopoly on the floor, only to end up rolling around laughing after a trumping competition. Or the times when they'd create their own singing and dancing routine to the likes of 'Bohemian Rhapsody'. They were like fire together.

Oh, he was so soft with her and she knew how to play him like a fiddle! When she was coming up to 14, she wanted a laptop. I was hesitant, unsure about exposing her too early to the internet – this was at a time when it wasn't so normal to give children their own tech devices.

Anyway, around Father's Day that June, Dave and Si had a slot at the BBC's *Summer Good Food Show* at the NEC in Birmingham and we all went there to support him. The night before, a load of us went out to dinner – James Martin was there, Simon, our friend Steve, some of the Hairy Bikers' team and a few people who were organising the show – and there must have been about 20 of us at the table all having a whale of a time.

Iza sidled over to Dave, gave him a hug, sat on his lap and handed him an envelope. Inside was a card to 'The Best Dad in the World' and a pair of socks saying the same. Well, well, well. I knew exactly what she was up to! Dave was so chuffed and he turned to me and said, 'Tomorrow, please go and buy her that laptop.' Attagirl.

Iza has always had the confidence to go her own way and be entirely at ease in any situation – another quality she shared with Dave. From the off she was comfortable in the entertainment and foodie worlds Dave was part of and she'd quite happily chat to anyone backstage at the big arenas while Dave and Si were out front, doing their thing – from Irish baker Paul Rankin to Gordon Ramsay's mum or Gino D'Acampo.

On many occasions the boys would film in our house, or we would travel at weekends to wherever Dave and Si were working, so Iza got to know the tricks of the TV trade and she completely understood the Bikers' humour and dynamic. It made her the perfect candidate to work on their social media channels for a few years and she enjoyed adding another string to her bow.

She also had no qualms about coming home from university for the first time to announce, 'I'm now a vegetarian, I don't eat meat anymore.' What a blow for Dave! He was crestfallen.

'What?!' he replied, incredulous. 'I go all around the world finding recipes and we have all this exceptional food in our house and you're saying you won't be eating what I cook? That's outrageous!'

But guess what? It only made their relationship stronger, because Dave learned a different way of thinking and understood that Iza's decision came from her compassion for living and breathing things. Whenever she was home from that day on, he'd create healthy feasts for the family with plenty of green salads and separate bowls of carbohydrates and meats so that, veggie or not, we could add whatever we liked to our plates. He respected her choice and was proud of her determination to stick to her guns.

Iza had gone on to achieve 12 GCSEs, which I think is incredible for a student whose first language was not English. She nailed her A levels too and then her degree in Art at Manchester Metropolitan University. Dave and I were bursting with pride at the sight of her in the graduation robe, throwing her hat up in the air! What a fine young lady she'd become, ready to take on life and make it her own.

Sergiu, my son, is also an extremely hardworking person. After arriving in Barrow-in-Furness in 2008 having completed his exams in Romania, he worked throughout the summer in an Italian restaurant and in October 2008 started a degree in computer science at Aberdeen's Robert Gordon University. He was an adopted Scotsman by the time he finished five years later and at his graduation ceremony we all admired this young man from Transylvania receiving his certificate dressed in a kilt!

When writing his dissertation in his final year, Sergiu had expressed an interest in following up his studies with a master's degree to combine his computing knowledge with his passion for cars, having grown up watching Formula 1 on television with his father. Dave did a bit of scouring the internet and discovered that Oxford Brookes University offered an MSc in automotive sport engineering and were holding an open day that weekend. We made it a family trip and had a great time visiting the school's workshops – incomprehensible to me but thrilling for the boys – and when I spotted Dave and Sergiu sharing knowing glances, I quickly understood where this was heading. Sergiu wasn't going to do the year-long master's, he was signing up for the full four-year degree course.

He graduated with distinction, won a prize for a business plan he created and went straight to work at the Renault Alpine Formula 1 team – Sergiu and Dave's dream! The conversations between them were something else, so technical and passionate. I didn't fit in because I knew next to nothing about circuits, aerodynamics or the tyres of a racing car. Sergiu and Dave would watch the race build-ups, making educated predictions, suffering together when it didn't play out as they'd forecast and naughtily sharing a cigar (hoping I wouldn't catch them) when it did.

In 2023 Sergiu would bring us to Silverstone, taking Dave on the Pit Lane Walk ahead of the F1 race, where all the celebrities and VIPs get to go. That was golden for Dave, who had watched it all on TV for years and had long aspired to get there one day himself. What a privilege for him. Mind you, when Sergiu told us he wanted to get his motorbike licence, Dave went into full-on dad-panic mode, as he understood better than anyone the enthusiasm for engines and vehicles, but also knew about the dangers.

Dave always wanted to do right by the kids. He never tried to replace their father but every decision we took as a couple included the two of them, and as much as Dave and I loved our time together as a couple, we could never separate ourselves completely from the unit that was our family. Wherever we went just the two of us, he would always say, 'Oh, we have to bring the kids here some day!'

Would Dave have been a different father if he'd had his own biological children? I'm certain the answer to this question is no. He loved Sergiu and Iza dearly and took every opportunity to tell them that. Those feelings were reciprocated and will be forever.

* * *

As the Hairy Bikers expanded, so Dave outgrew the small kitchen on Piel Street and it became obvious that we needed to extend. We had some space in the courtyard so while he was away filming in 2009, I oversaw the building work. All the dust and the discomfort of living in a house undergoing a renovation was largely (and conveniently for him) missed by

Dave and I had to figure out how to hire and fire people, who to trust and who to avoid. It was a learning curve for sure.

The effort was all worth it in the end when our beautiful kitchen was complete and Dave was in his element with his new workspace, not just for the possibilities it offered but also because it was a symbol of the Hairy Bikers' success story so far.

The boys were so dedicated and tireless – with every series came long negotiations, creative juices and a lot of planning. On several occasions, and for one reason or another, those plans did not come to fruition but Dave and Si both had such high hopes for the brand and I could always feel his excitement when he came home from meetings about taking it to the next level. He was so trusting that he could never fathom the idea of it not being successful, but such is life, sometimes other people would let them down and promises would prove empty which was hard for him to take.

I believed in him wholeheartedly and never doubted that the two of them had something special, but there were times when I watched Dave setting off on the bike at two in the morning in apocalyptic rain to travel to wherever they were shooting that day and I worried. Don't forget, travelling on a bike is only poetic and bohemian when the weather is fine. When it's not and your clothes are heavy with rain and you can't see anything in front of you, it's hard, physical work and it can be treacherous.

Dave and Me

While they were filming *The Hairy Bikers' Food Tour of Britain* in the winter of 2008–9, Dave arrived home, exhausted, freezing cold and soaked through his leathers to the skin. He couldn't get out of them because the fabric had stiffened from him being in the same position on the bike for so long and I had to put him in a hot bath, fully clad in his leathers, so they could soften enough for us to peel them off. It wasn't unusual for precious weekends together to be written off because once the adrenaline had stopped running through his veins, his body would just give up and he'd come down with a debilitating cold. Much about the television industry is not glamorous in the slightest.

Personally, I thought they worked too hard, but Dave would say, 'Darling, this is the work to build the brand and that means making some sacrifices along the way.' It wasn't just about building a brand, of course. It was about fulfilling dreams and experiencing the world – Dave loved the work he did and what he and Si were creating together. And I loved watching him on the TV although I never thought of myself as having a celebrity for a partner. We were spoiled by the food he made and the stories he came home with, but our life as a couple and a family was all very normal.

I was also keen to work myself and to start earning a living again, although with Dave's unpredictable schedule, finding something to fit around the school runs was a challenge. That's why I decided to go back to the first craft I learned, having worked in that 'sweatshop' clothes factory for 13 years, and I opened a little workshop at home, doing clothing and soft furnishing alterations and repairs.

Dave took me to Birmingham to a sewing exhibition and I picked out a new sewing machine. Dave, as ever, wanted me to have the best tools possible and he had to persuade me because I wasn't mentally prepared to spend the amount of money he was suggesting. He eventually convinced me to allow him to pay the equivalent of a car for a top-of-the-range Pfaff machine which became my new baby, serving me for the next 15 years and helping me create some beautiful garments. I picked up jobs for local shops and gradually my little business started to flourish.

I kept it going for a few years until the Hairy Bikers were so in demand that Si hired a PA and I came on board to help Dave with organising his diary, logistical arrangements and taking care of the finances and paperwork. Stepping into this new world was unnerving at first and I felt awkward, different and inadequate, I had to learn how to mask all that discomfort and thankfully it was never something that Dave picked up on. Over time I learned to embrace the things that made me different and use them to my advantage, and a lot of that was down to Dave.

'You go, girl,' he'd say. 'You've got this, Lil.'

I'd say the only blight on our life on Roa Island was the behaviour of a rather tiresome neighbour who we shared access with and whose nonsense Dave had been suffering long before I turned up. For the purposes of this book and to protect his identity, I'll call him Mr Neighbour – he was the sort of person who managed to fall out with everyone and there weren't many people on the island who had much time for him.

He drove Dave potty.

'Bloody Neighbour,' he'd fume at the latest trivial issue he'd chosen to cause conflict over. Dave only ever referred to him by his surname.

Mr Neighbour always had a bee in his bonnet about something and could be verbally abusive – he'd talk about me and Iza as being 'the immigrants' but I refused to let him get to me. My policy with Mr Neighbour was not to become enraged by his constant state of indignation, but instead to kill him with kindness. We had to live alongside him, after all. So I always remained cordial.

When we started to consider selling the house on Piel Street, we didn't want to have a neighbours' dispute hanging over us, so I made it my business to resolve the differences once and for all. We had a shared-access driveway, owned 50:50 between us and Mr Neighbour and which ran along the side of our house to our garage. It was in a terrible state, full of potholes and in desperate need of repair – besides anything else, I knew we couldn't put our place on the market until this problem was solved. Dave had washed his hands of Mr Neighbour and wouldn't have anything to do with him, so I stepped into action and asked him to come round for a chat.

'We've got a buyer interested in the house who happens to be a lawyer,' I said, telling a little fib. 'And I expect he'll give you a hard time over this drive if he moves here, so surely it's better that we deal with this now? It'll enhance the value of your property too, and so everybody will be happy.'

By some sort of a miracle he agreed to going halves on getting the drive relaid. Job done. On our last day there, as we were clearing everything out to move into the new place, there was a knock on the door. I was surprised to see Mr Neighbour standing there.

'I just wanted to say goodbye,' he said. 'And to thank you very much for being so nice to me.' Then he kissed my hand. Dave was in the background, steam coming out of his ears! I'm not quite sure what was going on there, but to me it seemed sincere and I appreciated his gesture. Mr Neighbour probably hadn't had much kindness in his life because of the way he treated other people, but I suspect his anger came from something else way back in his past. Issues that he never resolved.

In the end, we lived on Piel Street for nearly four years – while there were things we adored about the island, we had decided that a move closer to Barrow town would be best for all three of us. We loved our house, but the windows faced directly onto the street and we'd often get passers-by staring in through the curtains. Sometimes their faces would actually be pressed against the glass! One evening while we were eating, I'd waved someone in as a joke and she took it seriously, knocking on the front door to come in. To our amusement, when Dave opened the door, this lady stepped over the threshold very confidently saying she'd been invited.

As well as the need for somewhere with a little more privacy, we also wanted to be closer to Iza's school so we could save time on the daily travelling to and from there. So, while Dave was away biking and filming, I'd started house hunting on my own – another first for me. Whenever he came home from his travels, I'd fill him in on my discoveries and we would talk over our various options. By now it was 2010, the Hairy Bikers had several series, books, a couple of Christmas specials and a live tour under their belts and it meant we had a budget that would allow us a house a bit bigger than the one we were leaving behind.

This was simultaneously exhilarating and scary for me. Back in Romania you live in the same house for your whole life and are tied to the land and to your property, yet here I was, changing homes twice in the space of a few years.

Over the months I must have viewed about 50 properties within the Barrow and Ulverston areas, but there was always something that wasn't quite right. Until I found the Roman house. It was a semi-detached Victorian beauty on the most well-known road in Barrow. It was close to Iza's school and set back from the road, with spacious car parking at the front and a garden to the rear. Best of all, when I told Dave, who was away filming *The Hairy Bikers' Cook Off*, the boys' biggest series yet with 40 episodes commissioned, he started laughing out loud on the phone, remembering that in his teenage years the house was known as 'the local knocking shop'.

Apparently all the kids used to climb on the fences intrigued as to what might possibly be going on inside and the idea of owning that house tickled Dave. It had a pub in the cellar which, way back in time, had been quite an attraction in the town because it stayed open long after the local bars had shut for the night. I suspect the questionable reputation was more connected to that rather than anything more unsavoury, although Dave would often say wistfully, 'If only these walls could talk ...'

The new place was another renovation job and so I took on a building project all over again. The difference this time was that we hadn't yet sold the house on Roa Island and therefore didn't have to live among the chaos. There were a few snags, however. After the purchase of the new house had gone through, I'd encountered a number of obstacles because I wasn't 'the wife'. Trying to switch utilities to the new address and paying various tradespeople was a nightmare as we weren't married and I got so annoyed with the situation that I decided to take action.

I should say that we were already engaged in all but name at this point after Dave had called me at midnight on his 50th birthday during my first week in Barrow when he was working away.

'Sweetheart, turn to your right and open the drawer,' he'd said. Inside was a box with a beautiful, antique diamond and sapphire engagement ring and it felt very romantic, although he never actually proposed. Marriage was a technicality to us; our love was stronger than conventions and being partners in life was enough. But now I was taking matters into my own hands. I made a few phone calls and the next time Dave came home from filming, I informed him that we were to be married on 8 January 2011.

That was in precisely six weeks.

'WHATTTT?!'

You heard it, Mr Myers!

The Wedding Ring

2 October 2024

Today I'm tidying the tall, dark, wooden chest of drawers in our bedroom where Dave kept his socks, belts, ties and his prized collection of colourful handkerchiefs. It's the hankies I'm keen to take a look at. I'm planning to repurpose some of them into embroidered decorative leaves for the poppies I'm crocheting for the forthcoming Remembrance Sunday.

Dave was always so regimented with his handkerchiefs, keeping them all perfectly pressed, picking one out each morning, unfolding it with a theatrical shake before squashing it into his pocket. If I ever questioned the point in ironing them when they were destined only to be crumpled, he would reply, 'Because I'm worth it!'

They had a practical use too, when going on work trips. He'd pack one for each day he was going to be away and then use them to calculate how long he had left on the road. He stored them all in the top drawer which I have to raise myself onto the tips of my toes to reach, but there they are.

All neatly folded into little squares, just how he liked them. I run my hand over the soft cotton.

But hold on … there's something else here too. I can feel it nestling between one of the piles. My breath catches. Dave's wedding ring. I'd thought this had been lost forever. I'd noticed it wasn't on his finger a few weeks before he passed and had turned the house upside down trying to find it. I'd called the hospital asking if he'd maybe left it there. I'd searched the car in case he'd dropped it during one of our journeys to appointments.

Dave racked his brains but couldn't remember where or when he'd last seen it and I was gutted for him because he was so cross with himself. Gutted for me too, that this symbol of our union had seemingly vanished. I can see now what happened. His fingers were so thin towards the end and the ring must have slipped off without him noticing while he was reaching into the drawer one morning for a handkerchief.

How I wish I could tell him that I've found it and it's safe now.

This simple gold band was one of the very few pieces of jewellery Dave ever wore. Funnily enough, it wasn't the first wedding ring he managed to lose. That one – the original – was bought along with mine from an antique shop in Bratislava back in December 2010. We were there on my birthday and after buying our rings, Dave had booked a limo to take us to a 'floating' restaurant on the Danube called UFO, which offered awesome panoramic views of the Slovakian capital.

That ring went AWOL three years into our marriage when Dave was performing an escapology routine on stage in Hull. As you do. Sometimes it's only when I write these things down that I realise how crazy our life together could be. But yes, part of the boys' *Hairy Bikers: Larger Than Life* theatre tour in 2013 involved Dave, dressed in a pair of gold hotpants (because, what else?), being locked in chains from which he had 30 seconds to escape. While trying to free himself, the wedding ring had fallen off his finger and although Dave, Si and the stage tour crew did everything possible to locate it, they had no success. He even went on social media appealing for the public's help, only to have a reply from someone saying, 'You should go to the pawnshop, you'd have more luck there.'

He didn't have the heart to tell me on the phone, but confessed the next time he came home and said how odd it felt without it on his finger. I went out that same day to buy a replacement and it's this one I've just found, having believed he'd lost it for the second time.

I can feel my legs start to shake, so I take a seat on the edge of the bed and my mind spins off, remembering our sensational wedding day. Dave was so dashing in his kilt. We'd never actually discussed getting married until the day I told him it was happening in six weeks' time, and Dave had gone into a panic as he always did when there was a surprise unfolding and the decision was not his.

'You need to call my agent and book the date off,' he said.

I already had.

In fact, I had it all figured out. One of my colleagues, Terry, was a registrar and would conduct the service, and my parents were booked in to visit from Romania, although they had no idea of my plans.

Dave tried to pitch in by hiring a party planner he'd found online, but I think she was more used to organising kids' birthdays, so I had to let her go and took over everything myself. It didn't faze me. I even made my own wedding dress. The night before the big day, my friends in Barrow had organised a lively hen do for me in the basement bar of our new house on Abbey Road, complete with a gargantuan Hairless Hairy Biker 'stripper' (who turned out to be the security guard at the local job centre) wearing a red bra and fishnets. There was also a hairless Elvis impersonator who ended up losing his wig and most of his clothes, too. At one point, he had one of my more tipsy friends in a fireman's lift over his shoulder.

Dave had taken his stag do on a train from Barrow to a pub about half an hour away in Foxfield in the Lakes. When the 40 of them arrived back into Barrow station later that night, the police were waiting because someone had reported them for being too rowdy on the train. Busted before his big day! That wasn't a big enough warning sign for them to call it a night though ... Put it this way, my son and nephew, who had been with the stag party, arrived home at four in the morning. We were getting married at twelve.

Dave and Me

On 8 January 2011, Dave and I were married at the town hall in Barrow-in-Furness in front of 150 guests. The room was beautifully decorated with flower arrangements in different shades of white and a string quartet played beautiful music all day. Si did a speech, as did Dr Dave who used a PowerPoint presentation (very typical of Dr Dave who is always all or nothing!) featuring pictures from over the years.

Many more joined us for the evening do at the 99 Club and there were about 400 of us partying the night away with scrumptious food provided by Barrow's Thai community. We had a 20-kilogram wedding cake made by Slattery in Manchester which was covered in 100 white chocolate roses, and a Blues Brothers tribute band who had everyone up on the dancefloor the whole night long. We'd put a fair amount of money behind the bar but the guests had obliterated it by the time I got there myself and I had to buy my own drink! What a party it was …

I'm staring at the lost (now found) ring, comforted by the thought that it still holds Dave's biological residue and is keeping another connection to him open and alive.

I've been thinking about connections a lot. When we lose someone, pain is the only visceral emotion that physically connects us to them. In fact, we often *crave* it because it's a link between the full life we once had and the enormous empty space left after loss. Anything to fill that void and re-trigger the feelings that once were our normal state.

It's a hardwired biological need, rooted in our evolutionary history, and means the difference between life and death, success or failure, belonging or separation. Consciously, we know how the pain erodes us and we long for it to end. But unconsciously we want it to continue because if we stop feeling it, we fear the emotional bond goes too.

My own interpretation of this is structured around making a big, brave decision to stay connected by honouring the beauty of the relationship. Within the realms of our individual personal circumstances, we all – and I say this lovingly – have that choice. When we put our attention towards something our minds and deeds will follow, whether it's positive or not. If you don't take some sort of conscious action to step out of the pain, you can remain engulfed in it, eaten up by guilt, caught in a loop.

A good analogy for this involves a motorbike, aptly enough. When you're driving a motorbike and you have to go around something, it's your head and your hands that move first. The bike then follows.

By making a decision to focus on memories of good times and by moving your thoughts and attention towards the positive, your body learns to associate these uplifting feelings with your loved one.

I have used Emotional Freedom Tapping to help relieve myself of negative thoughts, taking in pressure points at the top of the head, the eyebrows, in the corners of the eyes, under the eyes, on the mouth, chin, collarbone and under the arm. I identify what is driving the fear and assess the level of anxiety it's causing on a scale of zero to ten. Then I choose a statement that addresses the fear – for instance, 'Even though I feel stress, I accept myself completely' – and start tapping on the pressure points in sequence, moving down the body, staying aware of my anxiety levels as I'm doing so and taking note of where they are on the scale as they begin to subside.

It might go down from an eight to a six, then to a five until everything calms and it becomes clear that it's within my power to bring those levels down – therefore I can control how I react and determine where my mind goes. It doesn't happen easily at the beginning and it takes effort to get going, but one step at a time, one thought after another and you will start to make a shift. And once you've found that state of contentment, you can make another decision to stay there.

This ring is helping me do that now as I remember the best day with the best people. Love and happiness. Dave swinging me around the dancefloor to Scorpions' 'Rock You Like a Hurricane' and enjoying the party of his life.

I'm smiling now. But my god, I'd swim oceans to have him back. Anything to erase the last few years of illness and grief. I place the band on the fourth finger of my right hand and promise never to take it off.

Chapter Six

Life and Soul

That cake is lighter than an angel's fart

I've heard it said that people often fall into one of two camps. There are thermometers – those who reflect the temperature of the room they're in. They blend in and adapt to their surroundings but lack the power to change them. And then there are thermostats. They are the ones who set the temperature of the room, bringing everyone else along with them. They create the atmosphere, generate the energy and are the people we gravitate towards.

Dave was, most definitely, a thermostat.

He had the power to lift a whole room just by being in it; it was all so effortless for him because he thrived on company and connection. Wherever Dave and I were living, our house was always full. Buzzing with life. Friends, family, neighbours, colleagues and even passing acquaintances – there were always people around. We both loved entertaining and he preferred to host, quite simply because being on home turf meant he'd be in control of the menu! Food was sacred to Dave and that was his happy place.

He'd make friends wherever he went, whoever they were and whatever the circumstances – in bars, on trains, during intervals at the theatre, without fail Dave would end up engaged in conversation. He'd go to the pub and come back with a gardener he'd got talking to.

'Lil, you said you needed some help in the garden. This is the man who can help!'

And said man would stay for a drink and further chat.

Nights out rarely ended at closing time. After last orders, the fun would continue back at our place into the early hours, with music, dancing, the drinks free-flowing and Dave holding court with his stories. Thanks to his passion for adventure, he had a bottomless barrel of colourful tales which he'd bring to life with descriptive language, telling the story with his whole body. Dave was always so animated as he recounted his escapades. He certainly knew how to put on a party and wherever we went, he'd bring the fun, the unexpected twist, the spark, always looking for ways to create memorable moments.

The very first restaurant he ever took me to in Paris was right by the Seine and called Lapérouse. He'd read a story about the mirrors in the building which bore hundreds of scratch marks from, according to legend, the mistresses testing the authenticity of the diamonds bought for them by their royal lovers. Dave loved that story, so that's why we went!

Another time in Paris, we were in a taxi on our way to one restaurant when he suddenly told the driver to stop the car.

'Truffles,' he said to me. 'I can smell truffles!'

His highly trained nose had caught a whiff from the open window of the taxi, so he had the cab stop in central Paris and we got out so he could follow the smell to find where it was coming from. He cancelled the original place, got a table at this new one and enjoyed the truffles he'd sniffed out at 50 paces.

There was no such thing as a run-of-the-mill holiday with Dave. His busy schedule rarely allowed us to make many plans far in advance, so we didn't manage to get a honeymoon after our spontaneous January 2011 wedding. However, that summer he found himself with an unexpected three weeks off, so on the spur of the moment we booked a cruise, something that had been on both of our wish lists for a while.

We went online to have a shop around and in true Dave spirit he found the most extravagant holiday on offer, a Mediterranean experience with Cunard, which set sail from Southampton. Fabulous! We booked a suite, packed our bags and off we went, excited for the two and a half weeks ahead with planned stops in Cadiz, Barcelona, Catania and Dubrovnik, among others.

Our table in the sumptuous dining room was tucked away in a corner on the first night, but a member of staff recognised Dave and the following day, we found ourselves 'upgraded'. We were now in a prime spot right in the centre of the room with dining companions varying from politicians to businesspeople – all of whom knew how to have a good time.

At one of the neighbouring tables was the restaurateur John Tovey and his partner. Dave had admired John, one of the first celebrity chefs, for a long time so he was a little starstruck. And he couldn't believe it when John got up and came over to shake his hand. From that moment, the dynamic in the previously quiet, formal dining room completely changed and we had a ball where conversation flowed and people came over to say 'hello' and clink glasses. Each night, Dave, John and various others swapped colourful stories and became deeply engaged in discussions about food and the world of TV while sharing wine and deliberating intensely over what they were going to order for dinner. This was all under the watchful eyes of the other diners who would see what Dave was ordering and then ask Osman, the maître d', for the same dish.

The head chef came to say hello one night and invited us to visit the bowels of the ship the next day where Dave had a chat and a laugh with the crew – it turned out that the Hairy Bikers' programmes were part of the internal TV network offered to staff, and many stewards, bell boys, cleaners and kitchen porters recognised him and wanted pictures and a handshake.

Dave then served them lunch of a divine-smelling Philippine curry in their own cantina, as a way of thanking them for their hard work. At dinner that evening, he asked Osman for the same curry, although it was not on our menu. Osman happily obliged and then had to deliver the same off-menu dish to half of the dining room as well!

Naturally, Dave relished the social side of cruise life. While we were on board, he and I took part in the ship's version of *Ready Steady Cook* which was held on stage in the amphitheatre. We were on opposing teams and unfortunately I was on the losing side, which was no surprise. Dave was always winning. Although really, everyone in the room won too, because he made the contest so entertaining, sharing riotous tales and revealing behind-the-scenes Hairy Bikers' secrets as he cooked, to the delight of our fellow holiday-makers.

At times, I was just as guilty as Dave for instigating funny situations although, in my defence, he usually would be the bad influence nudging me to do so. A charity ball we attended one year had a week on a Caribbean island on the auction list which jumped right off the page to me.

'Go on, Lil!' said Dave, encouraging me to get involved in the bidding and then egging me on to go higher each time. What we didn't know (until I finally won it) was that this tiny, private island was two hours off the Nicaraguan coast and accessible only by dinghy. Oh well, we'd paid for it, so we'd better go. The island was no bigger than a football pitch and although we had a beautiful beach-front suite, we were the only guests on the site. In the daytime there wasn't much to do except enjoy the sun and sea, by night we'd watch the baby turtles hatch from their nests and find their way to water.

It was a gorgeous place, but Dave got bored with so little to do and asked one of the caretakers to take him fishing. While on the trip, he managed to impale his thumb on a rusty hook and they had to take him on a two-hour boat journey to the nearest jungle hospital to have it removed. This could only have happened to Dave. He came back after midnight, happy and full of morphine. And at least we lived to tell the tale.

We had some wild times, I can tell you …

For his 60th birthday in 2017, we took a bunch of friends, the kids and their partners over to Mallorca where a chef he'd worked with called Marc Fosh ran a Michelin-starred restaurant in a converted convent which had also been transformed into a five-star boutique hotel.

We went to a phenomenal place with a luxury spa, rooftop pool and enormous rooms. There were 14 of us and we ate a beautiful eight-course dinner with champagne followed by a birthday cake complete with 60 candles. Si hadn't been able to join us, but he'd arranged for a few bottles of wine to be brought to the table.

We all got appallingly drunk before heading back to the suite Dave and I were staying in where there was a huge terrace and a jacuzzi. Everybody stripped off and dived straight into the hot tub, drinking and laughing and being generally outrageous. By now it was about two in the morning and we were

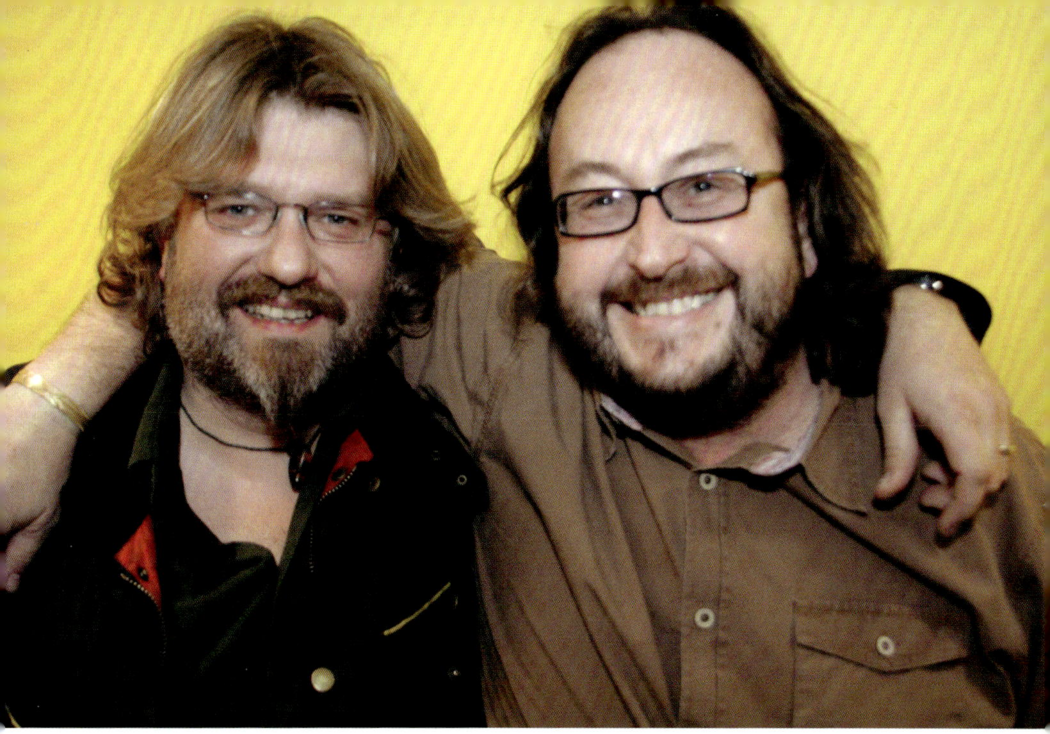

Si and Dave promoting their cookbook shortly after we met. Months later, I sewed a button on Dave's same shirt, making him tearful.

Myers Superior, Dave's custom-made motorbike which could raise the dead with the loud noise it made!

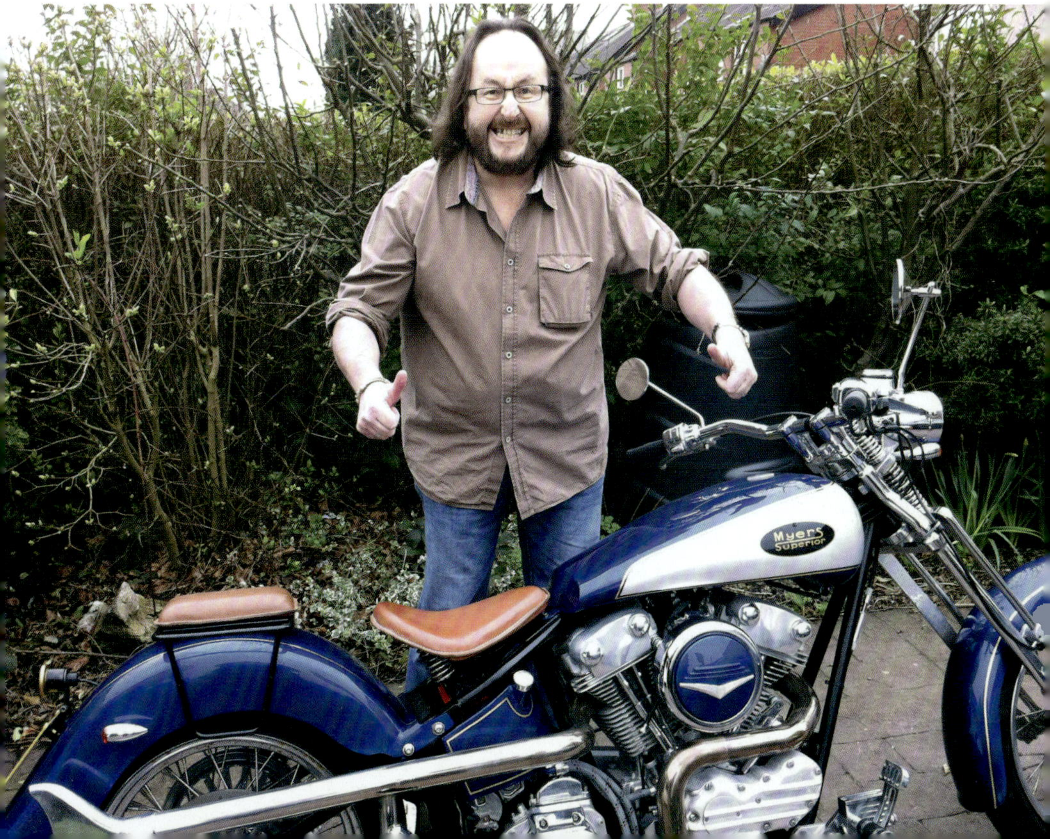

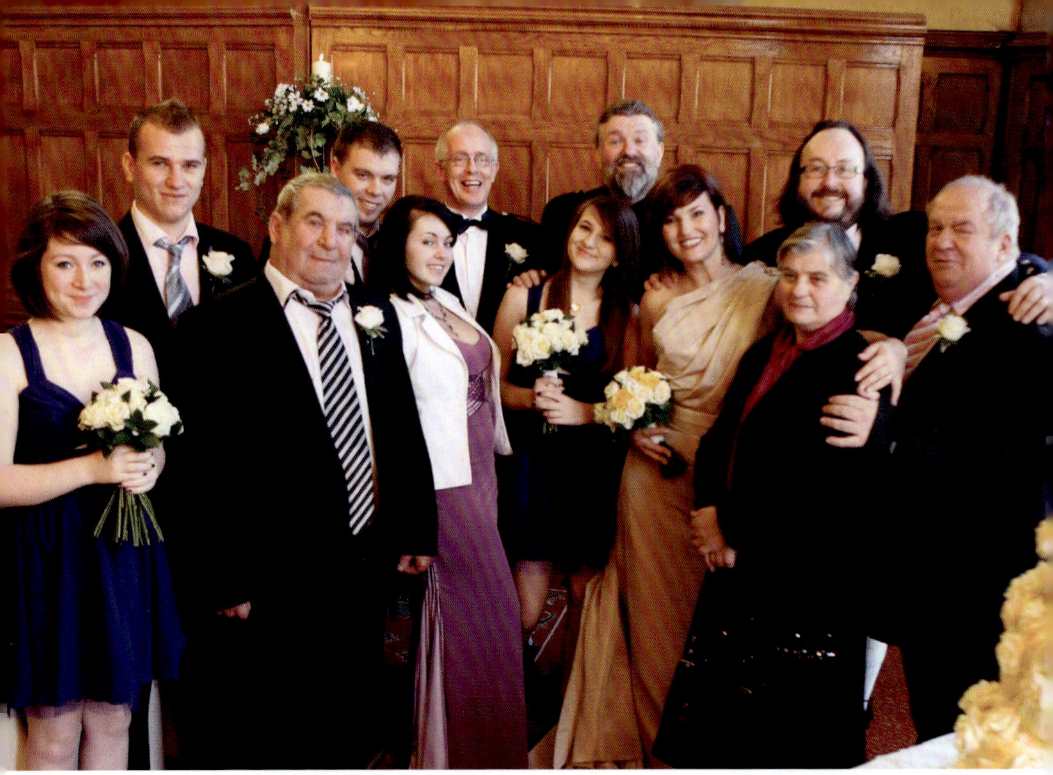

My family on our wedding day. We've since lost the two most important pillars, Dave and my dad. I held both their hands while they crossed the bridges and I feel so humbled and honoured.

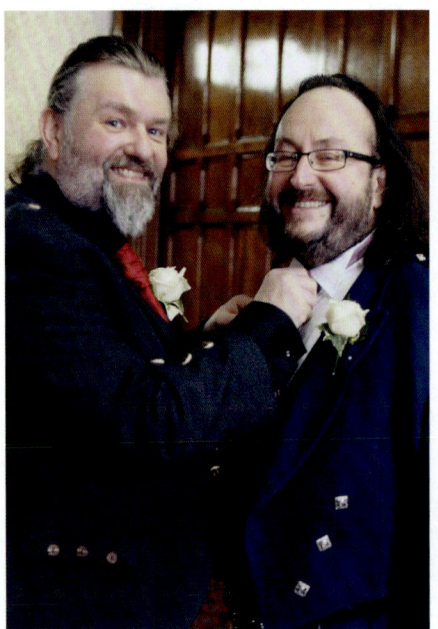

The two boys having an intimate moment just before we were wed.

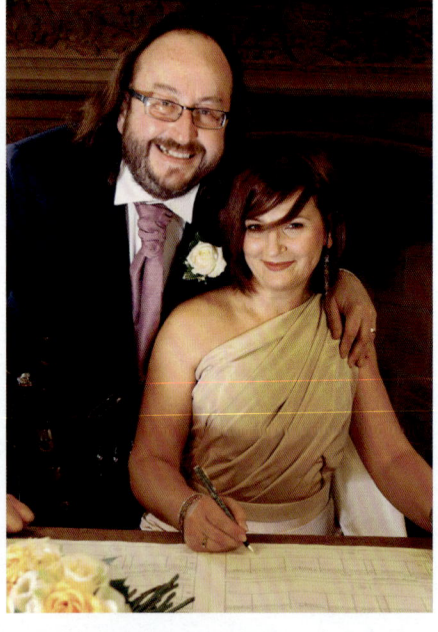

One of the very few photos of us from our big day, kindly taken by a guest and forwarded on to us.

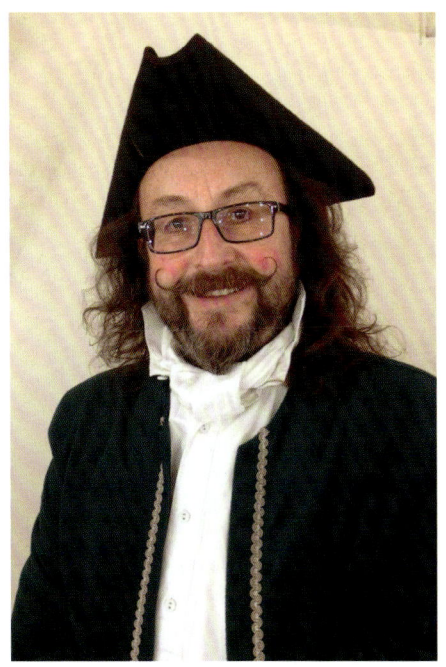

In Reading, where Dave played Baron Hardup in *Cinderella*. He kept the turn-up tache ever after.

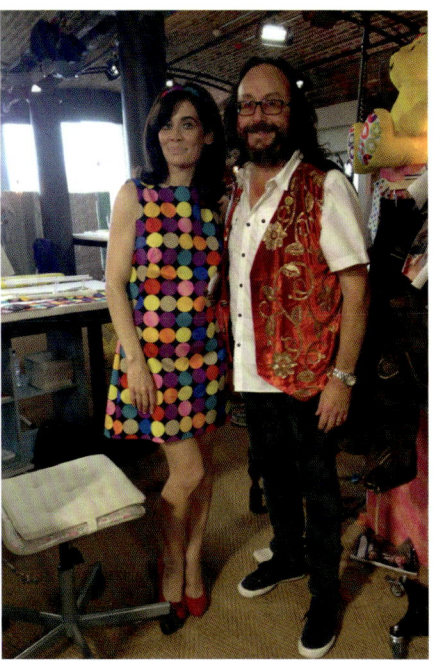

On *The Great British Sewing Bee*, with the sixties-style dress he made in four hours.

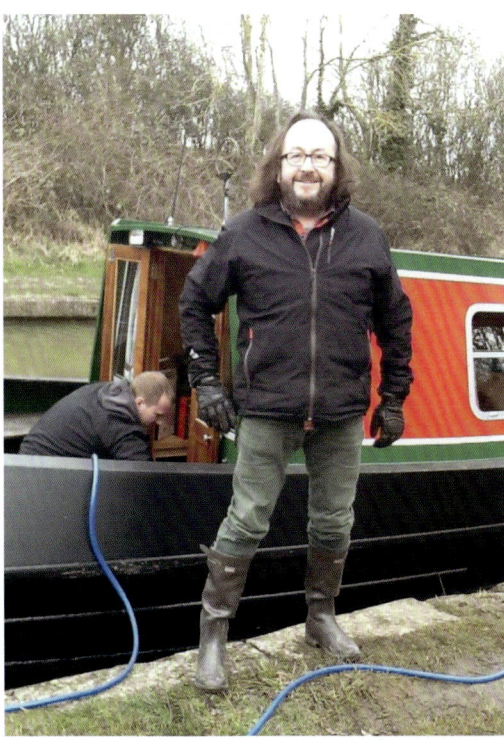

Our boating experiences were fantastic.

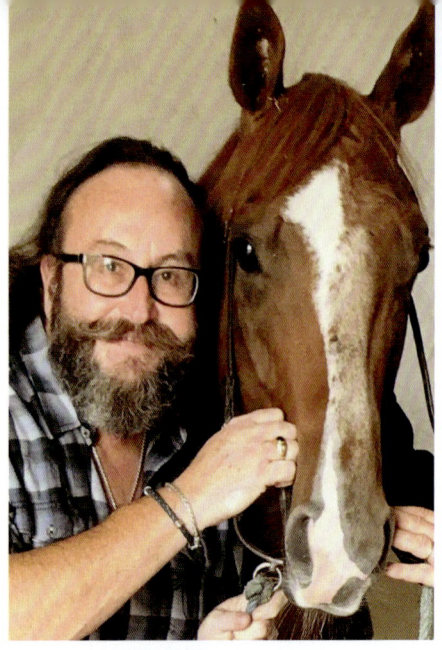
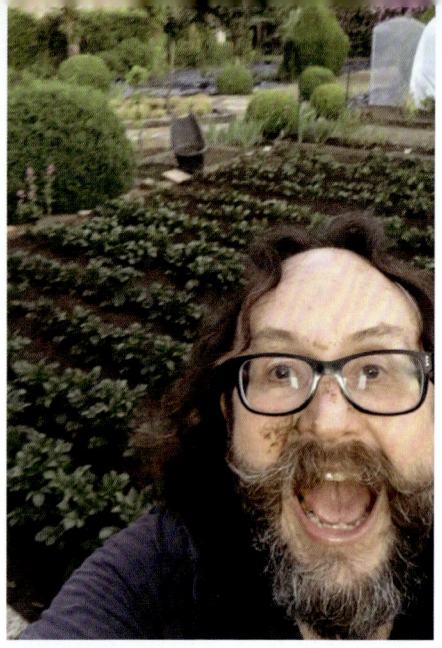

Dave and Tollie, before a race. He loved that horse so much!

My husband at his best, in the French veggie garden. One of my very favourite pictures of him.

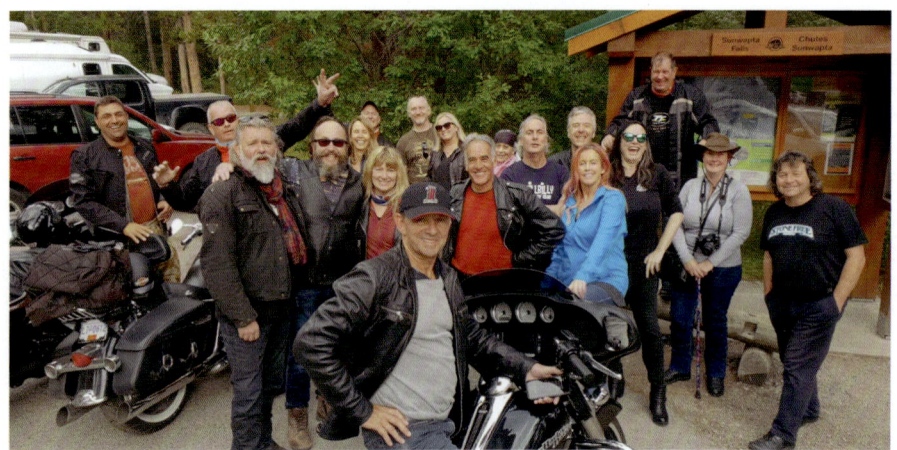

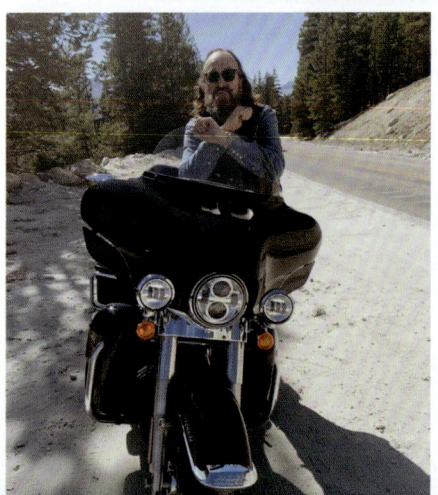

The Sons of Royalty on one of our epic motorbike journeys. We toured Europe, Canada and the States on Harley-Davidsons and raised more than £700,000 for the NSPCC.

Busted for 'endangering animal life' in Yosemite National Park!

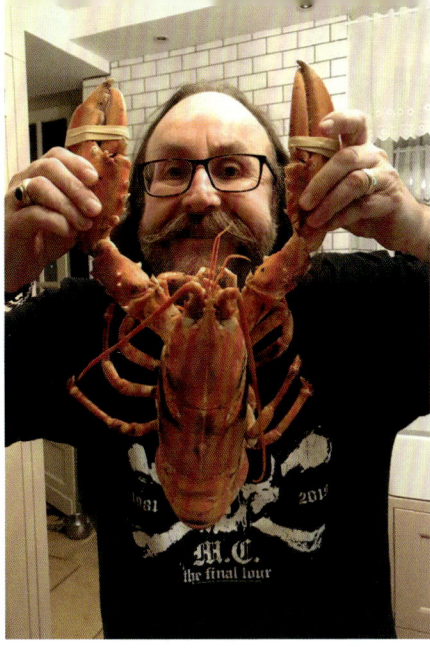

After buying a beautiful lobster-decorated serving platter, Dave needed to cook the perfect lobster and serve it on that plate!

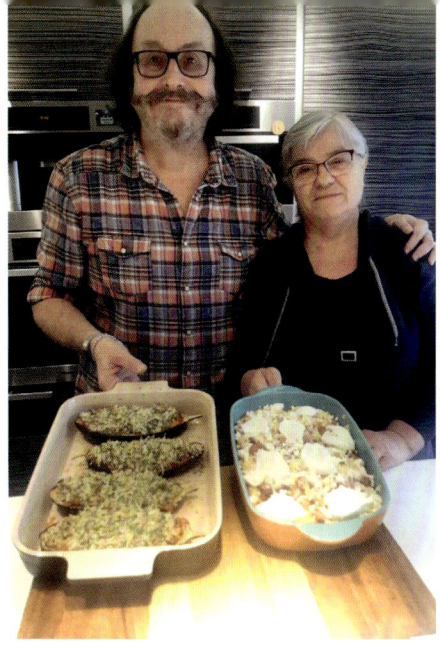

My mum and Dave were hilarious in the kitchen together. They could never agree on how to do anything ...

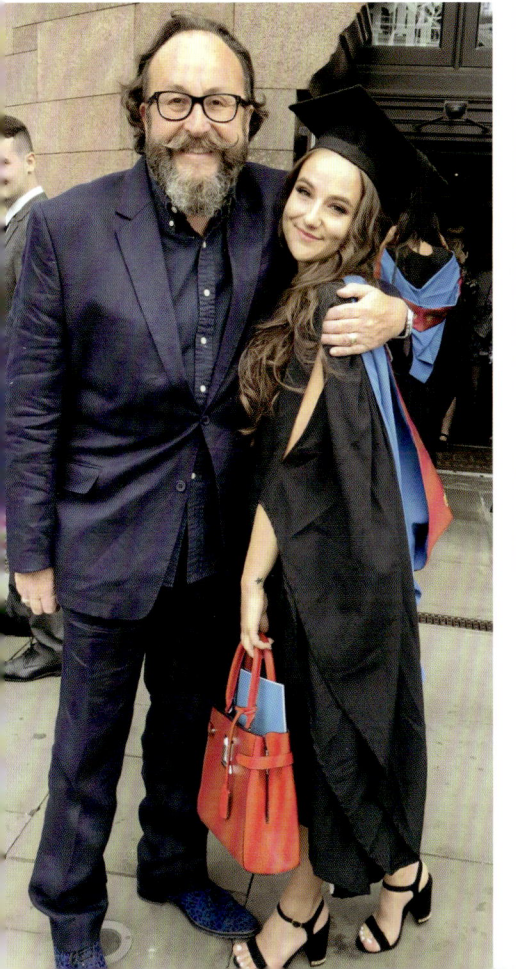

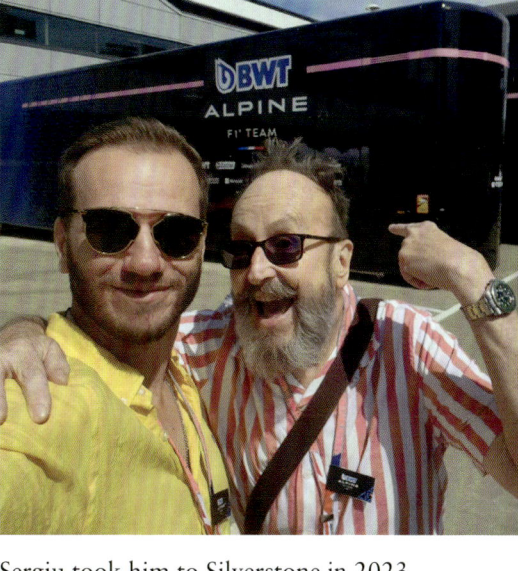

Sergiu took him to Silverstone in 2023. It had been his dream to do a Pit Lane Walk before an F1 race and finally that dream came true.

Proud Dave on Izabelle's graduation day.

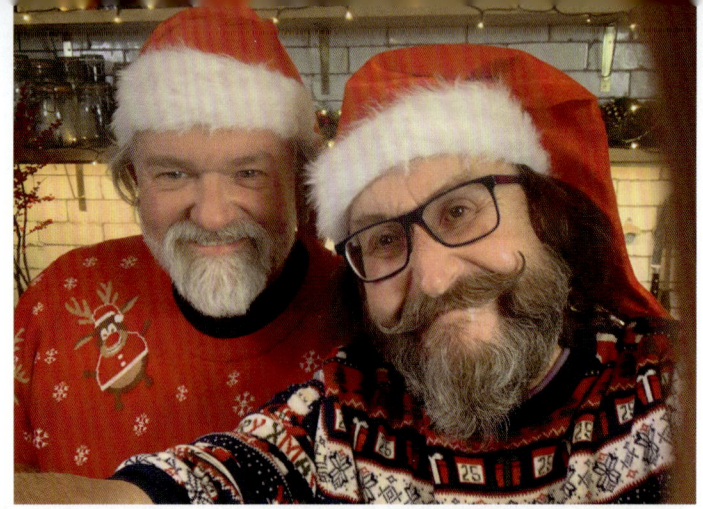

The wonderful
Christmas Dave.

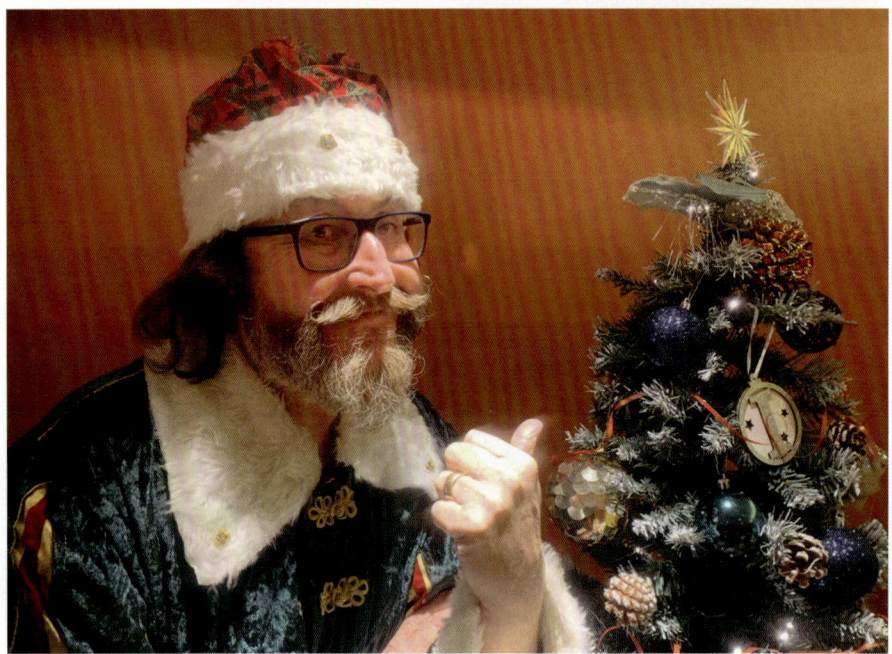

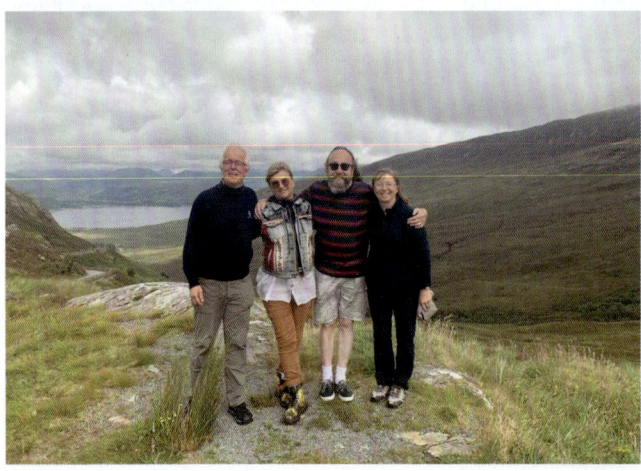

A visit up in
Scotland to see our
friends David and
Jane Easton.

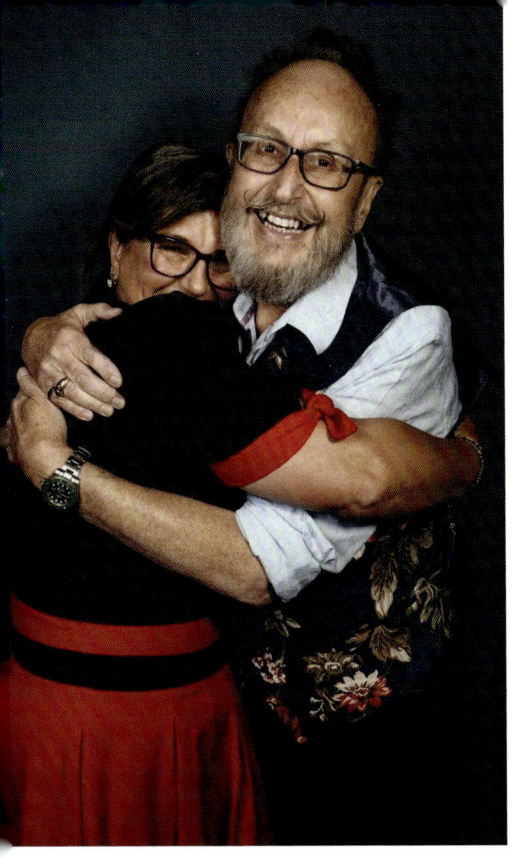

Our last picture together before Dave's health deteriorated.

Ahead of the last series, *Go West*, the boys meet their bikes for the first time. Dave's BSA Gold Star was very kindly donated by BSA for a charity auction and it fetched an impressive amount. It will be much loved by its new owner, Si Harrison.

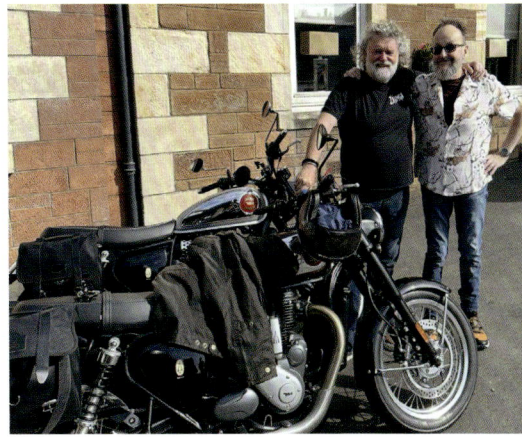

His 66th birthday was a chemo day. The wonderful nurses surprised him with a song and a cheesecake.

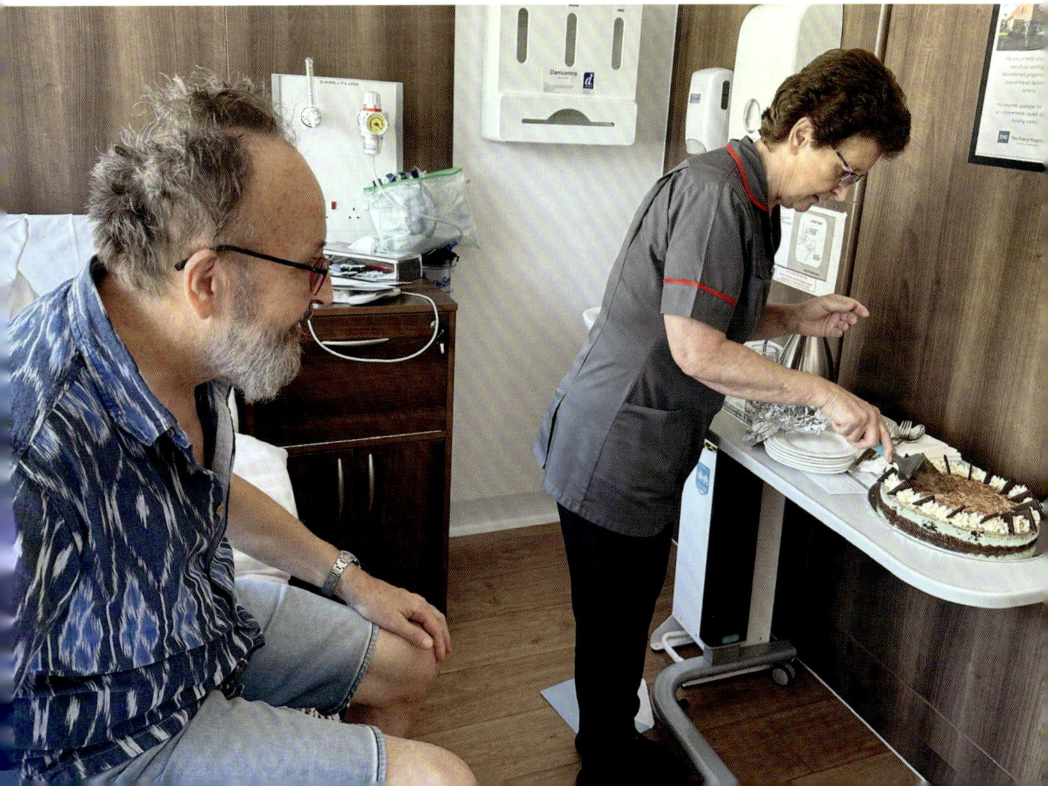

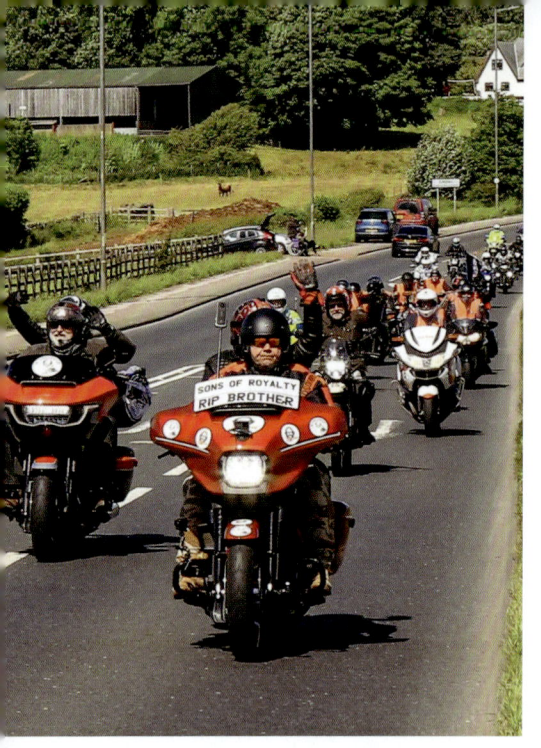

Dave Day 2024. I was a pillion on the first bike in the convoy with our friend Woody, who took the time and energy to organise the bike ride.

I was waiting to join the convoy at Knutsford Services.

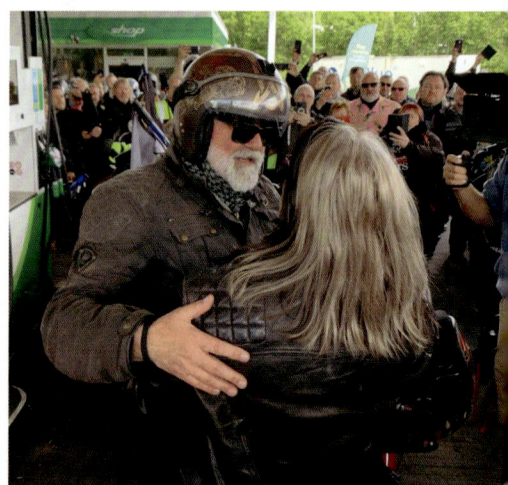

Barrow organised a wonderful hero's welcome for us.

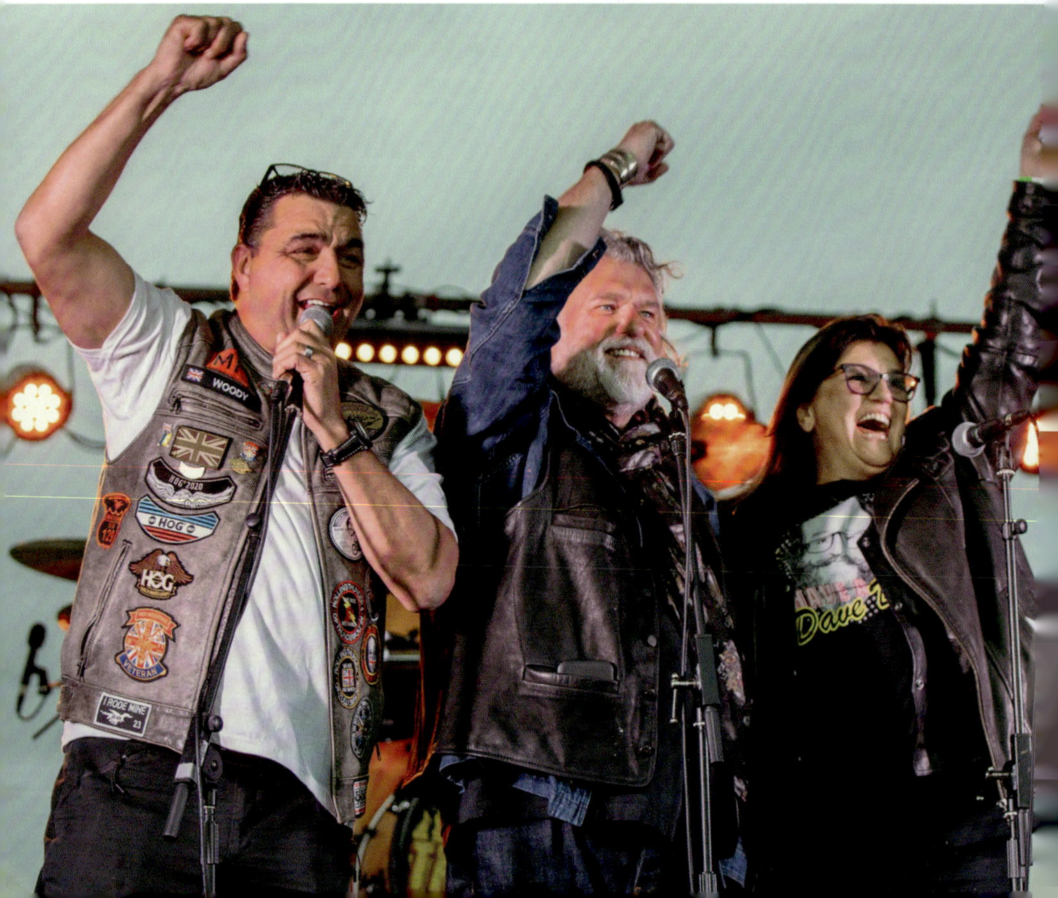

all far too carried away to notice the police on the roof of the building, frantically trying to get our attention to tell us to keep the noise down ... whoops.

Luckily for us, Dr Dave, who can drink anybody under the table and was therefore stone-cold sober despite having drunk the same as everyone else, spotted the cops. Unbeknown to any of the rest of us, he slipped away from the party, met with the officers and used a bit of the old Dr Dave smooth talk to calm the situation down.

Thank goodness for friends like him. The next day everybody was disgustingly hungover and had to do a lot of walking around the island to wear off the excesses of the night before.

* * *

Dave had a knack of drawing people in – his hunger for fun was infectious, transcending culture and language barriers, and this was never better demonstrated than when we were in Romania. It didn't matter that they didn't understand each other, my whole family loved Dave and he loved them right back.

During a trip one summer for my nephew's wedding, Dave was having such a great night ('thermostatting', you might say) that I couldn't persuade him to leave, even at six in the morning. It was his first experience of a Romanian wedding and he went at it full throttle, bopping about on the tables with the bride and taking part in a traditional dance with the men where they all put their hands on a neighbour's shoulders to form a circle and then make small stompy steps to the rhythm of a drum.

Speaking of wedding traditions, there was a point when Dave had a most bizarre moment completely by accident and which prompted much hilarity. There's an old Romanian custom that on the stroke of midnight, the groom's friends 'steal' the bride and spirit her away until a ransom – usually in the form of a crate of beer or a bottle of Jack Daniel's – is paid by the groom. The ransom negotiations are hard-fought and conducted by the groom's family which, as my nephew's godparents, should have included myself and Dave.

Anyway, Dave was dancing his socks off, away in his own little La La Land, when he saw the groomsmen making away with the bride and, not really knowing what was happening, he decided to tag along, squishing into the car with them. Sitting on the lap of one of the boys, he laughed, 'I'm sorry I'm so fat!' although none of them spoke English and so didn't understand what he'd said.

The 'kidnappers' drove for about a mile until they arrived at a bar and phoned to begin negotiations for the bride's safe return and I think that's when it dawned on Dave that he was in the wrong place. He was supposed to be back at the wedding, thrashing out a good deal to get the bride back – it was most unorthodox for the groom's family to take part in the kidnap itself …

It didn't really matter; everyone thought Dave was pure comedy and he'd had the time of his life. When we finally got home and I tried to undress him to put him to bed, I found his shirt collar had rubbed the skin behind his head until it bled – that's how much force he'd thrown into all the dancing and partying. Anyone who watched *Strictly* will know that Dave wasn't a dancer but give that man some tunes and a dancefloor and you'd be hard pressed to get him off it again! He slept for the whole of the next day, with the face of an innocent baby.

Dave always looked forward to our trips to Romania and my country became like a second home to him. The very first time he and I went there together as a couple, he swept my mum up in his arms, giving her a big hug and a kiss on both cheeks. And then he took my dad to the neighbouring pub.

Dad always had a secret wish to take his son-in-law to the pub. My ex-husband was teetotal and so my father's wish had not been fulfilled … but then along came Dave! They didn't speak the same language, but going for a beer together meant so much more than a conversation. They must have had a rip-roaring session in there because Dave ran out of money and they returned home with a debt to the landlady that I had to go round and settle the next day. When I was there, she told me what a funny night it had been, adding that Dave had paid for a round for everybody in the room while showing off pictures of the kids on his phone. And apparently he'd asked my dad for my hand in marriage. Of course, my dad hadn't understood one word and so the pub landlady, who spoke a little English, had translated for him. At least he asked my dad I suppose, because he never properly asked me! That was something that became a running joke between us.

Later that same week I witnessed another priceless moment between Dave and my dad. While I was there, I'd had to do the necessary admin to renew my passport, which was not a simple operation and involved obtaining various documents from different offices, then having to queue to have them processed. This was unusual for Dave who was used to having the postal service manage all that in the UK.

Once we'd been through all the rigmarole and got back to my parents' house, passport renewal all sorted, he and my dad went outside into the courtyard to sit on a couple of stools under a canopy of grapes. I was indoors cooking with my mum with the window open which meant I caught some of the surreal conversation between them. Dave in English and my dad in Romanian.

Dave: 'Oh, Vasile, Lil and I went to this office today for her passport ...'

My dad nodded. '*A, daaa, ploua mult pe la voi.*' (Oh yes, it rains a lot where you live.)

Dave: 'Yeah, I know ... it's such a nightmare to have to fill in all those papers in different offices!'

Dad: '*Aha, mai aveti si soare din cand in cand?*' (Ah, you have sunny days from time to time.)

Dave: 'And of course, wasting all that time in a queue.'

Dave and Me

Dad: '*Daaa, cred ca e destul de frig iarna la voi.*' (Yes, I believe your winters are cold.)

This went on for some time, both men listening very attentively to what the other had to say, nodding along and then replying in their own language about something completely unrelated. It was delightful to see them having such a man-to-man talk. I eventually asked them if they wanted me to translate and we all ended up in a fit of giggles, fully appreciating these moments together.

I think my dad and Dave had a deeper connection than a language could express. Both were hard workers who had earned people's respect by committing to their jobs, aware that others depended on their reliability. They had huge respect for each other, although my dad could never understand how a man could enjoy being in the kitchen. Nor how he could perform on a stage while dressed in a red sequin dress, as he saw Dave doing in one of my parents' later visits to the UK. But that's another story ...

Dave became very attached to Romania and looked forward to every trip. Knowing how important it was for their identity, we made sure Iza and Sergiu spent holidays there with family and old friends and we'd often accompany them. We also had their father, grandparents, aunties and friends visit us in the UK. One of Dave's favourite times of the year to be in Romania was over the Christmas holiday for the parties, celebrations and – you guessed it – the food!

In Eastern Europe, Christmas Day is when you visit family and friends, with every house offering *sarmale* and *salata de boeuf* on the table and *palinca* in the glasses. *Palinca* is a local fruit spirit which almost everyone who has an orchard brews at home and keeps in two-litre plastic bottles that originally contained mineral water. That means you have to be extra vigilant and double check what's in the bottle before taking a swig of the contents and Dave quickly learned this very valuable lesson. This stuff is lethal at 50 per cent alcohol, so it hits you like fire and makes you, ahem, 'merry' for a full day.

I once found Dave asleep under the Christmas tree in my parents' house, his head resting on a crate of beer after partying on the *palinca* with my cousins and having cooked a feast for 40 people. He'd had a great time that night getting to know everyone, 'Oh, another cousin, cheers! … Another uncle, cheers to you too!'

Dave used to have a lot of fun comparing the foods in each house we visited at Christmas and at the end of the 'competition' he'd officially declare who his favourite cook was. It was always Auntie Aneta's *sarmale* that took his first prize, just to tease my mum who would get in a huff. She wasn't really mad, though. My mum grew so fond of Dave and loved him like a son – she was an avid viewer of the Hairy Bikers on the Hungarian channel TV Paprika, although I don't think she understood much of what was going on. She just loved watching Dave do his thing.

Dave and Me

In 2012 he brought the TV crew back to Romania for a second trip, this time to film *Hairy Bikers' Bakeation*, which saw him and Si take on an epic 5,000-mile journey across Europe. Dave ended the episode filming with my family, declaring, 'I've managed to put my Romanian family on the BBC!' That footage is so precious to me. My dad, who we lost a few years later, is there toasting with Dave with a glass of *palinca*. My Uncle Ilie gifted the boys a bottle of his own brewed spirit, my mum together with Auntie Aneta baked beautiful cheese buns for everyone and my cousins Dan, Liviu, Petre, Florin and Lazar prepared a big barbecue for the party and all their families were present around the table.

Yes, Dave, you really did put your Romanian family on the screen!

* * *

Our annual trips away with the Sons of Royalty group were always jolly affairs and full of thrills and spills. We'd been introduced to them by Danny Bowes, the lead singer of Thunder – Dave and Si had met him through their Sunday radio show on Planet Rock and we formed so many incredible friendships on charity rides on Harley-Davidsons across Canada and the States. Each trip would usually end with a brilliant evening of fun featuring a prize-giving ceremony and a live Thunder gig.

One year we were riding through California's Yosemite National Park where the speed limit was five miles per hour, when Dave and I got stuck behind a queue of cars trying to park. A little impatient, Dave overtook one of the cars but was spotted by an eagle-eyed Ranger who followed and flagged us down.

This Ranger was not a happy chappy.

'You, sir, are a danger to nature and to people,' Dave was told very sternly.

'Oh, but I only overtook a car,' replied Dave.

'In our park it's illegal to do that.'

'Oh … I'm so sorry …'

The Ranger wasn't in the mood for accepting apologies and started making some calls, holding us there as he did so. All the other bikers in our group rode past us, amused at the sight of a Hairy Biker being collared by the law. After about half an hour, either bored by the process or feeling he'd made his point, the Ranger decided to let us go. On one condition.

'Sir, you have to promise me never to endanger wildlife again.'

Dave apologised profusely.

'I won't, officer, I hear you, officer. I'm sorry, officer.'

'OK, on your way.'

We somehow managed to hold in our giggles until we were out of the Ranger's sight and then we let it go, utterly helpless for laughing.

On another trip with the group, we rode 1,500 miles through Alberta and British Columbia, making a stopover in

Jasper where unfortunately the hotel was beyond grim and the food could only be described as brown sludge. They even managed to screw up the simple salad I'd ordered by dumping their trademark brown sludge on top of it. Dave's meal consisted of some type of unidentifiable meat and a pile of old boiled potatoes, which he couldn't bring himself to eat. This was also his birthday, so we'd been hoping for something a bit more special. Edible at the very least!

The only conceivable solution was to find the nearest pub and make our own party. This is where Dave always came into his own. The thermostat. We located a bar and after a few beers, two of our party got their guitars out, Si found a makeshift set of drums (AKA the pub's sick bucket) and together they accompanied Dave who performed the most uproarious dance solo to 'La Bamba'.

I've got the whole scene on video on my phone and it makes me laugh today as much as it did back then. Dave did everything with humour, never taking himself seriously, his only aim to entertain and have fun. I have many, many videos like that, all taken during moments of joy, laughter and happiness. When I watch them now, I struggle to comprehend that this fizzing ball of energy has been taken away, and that's why I don't believe for a moment that it's gone.

Dave's energy just continues, it lives on everywhere, even through the pages of this book. It's why I've included some of my favourite quotes from him at the top of every chapter, those marvellous turns of phrase that just tripped off the tongue for Dave. I want to keep that energy going to honour everything he did and who he was.

If I didn't interpret it in that way, I think I would die from crying.

The Photos

10 October 2024

I've been asked to send a journalist one of our wedding pictures to feature alongside an interview I've given about Dave. There have been many media requests since he passed and I am gaining confidence with the ones I choose to fulfil.

From a cupboard in my office, I dig out the big black box where I keep all the mementoes from our wedding day, a time capsule of memories including the planning file, receipts and press clippings from the newspapers who reported on our day. The box contains hundreds of pictures of happy moments captured by numerous different cameras. A myriad of smiling faces – people I can remember and many that I can't. Some of them have since departed and are deeply missed.

There aren't many at all of me and Dave, just the two of us. There are, however, mountains of me, Dave and Si. That became a running joke after the wedding when we realised that somehow Si had crashed every single photo of us newly-weds. Si was and still is a constant in my life and I knew they came as a package … I do wish I could find a picture without him in it, though!

I carry on searching, surely there must be one somewhere in here.

I come across a snap of Dave's old art teacher from Barrow Boys, the ever-dapper Mr Eaton, pulling some moves on the dancefloor. Shortly after I moved to the UK, Dave and I were walking in Ulverston looking for a nice place to stop for lunch and we bumped into Mr Eaton. It was the first time he'd met me and he said to Dave, 'Who is this lady? She's not from here, is she? I can see that from the bone structure of her face … I want to paint this face.' He was such a flamboyant character and we became good friends. He used to visit me, bringing bunches of flowers picked from his garden and taking me out to lunch. Our wedding would be the last time we saw him because he passed away a few weeks later. Lovely man.

It feels comforting, sifting through these photos and reconnecting to this happiness, being transported back to a time when we were joyous and healthy. When we had a life. Old photos are such irreplaceable things, they are bridges from the present to the past – a holiday, a favourite restaurant or even just Dave cooking in the kitchen doing what he did best. Precious moments.

Ah, here's darling, elegant Muriel who is, as usual, radiating kindness. She's looking at me in a family group photo and her husband, Les, Dave's cousin, is nearby with his shock of bright-white hair. Les looks very proud in the picture with his sons Phil and Malcolm, and their families. Dave used to tell me how much he'd admired Muriel when he was a boy and that she always had her hair immaculately styled. Well, she certainly looks the part in this picture!

Bridget, who is Les and Muriel's granddaughter, is the same age as Iza and it was a match made in heaven when the two girls met for the first time. Adorably, they started calling each other cousins. My daughter needed the security of an extended family and I have valued all their friendships immensely over the years.

Also in shot is Clare, who is Bridget's mum and Muriel's daughter-in-law. Clare's house was such a welcoming place to go for a party, and Dave and I always felt very at home there. Clare is also an excellent cook. Her son Angus is there in the group as well – Dave always said he was the handsome one in the Myers' clan.

Aw … now here's my family. Looking at my dad's face in this picture makes me happy. He adored Dave and cried the whole way while walking me down the aisle. Dad used to call him 'Davis' and my mum still writes his name as 'Dev'.

Despite the happy occasion, my parents are a bit lost in this picture, out of their comfort zone, intimidated by not understanding the language and not knowing many people at the party. In the same photo are Sergiu and Iza and one of my nieces from Romania who had seen ladies wearing feathers on their fascinators for the first time and innocently asked: 'Why do the women here wear their chickens on their heads?'

So many pictures to go through.

Here's one of the jolly gang from the Isle of Man. Steve, Jenny, Nigel and Nikki. Steve and Nige are wearing the Manx tartan and you can tell just from their faces that these are people who know how to have a good time! Dave met Steve on the Isle of Man during the TT Races around the same time he met me. They became partners in crime for many a caper, both passionate about food, partying and making people laugh. The key ingredients as far as Dave was concerned.

Which brings me to two more cheerful faces, Rory and Wendy McClure, mayor and mayoress of Barrow at the time of our wedding. They were our neighbours on Abbey Road and we spent many days and nights with them having fun. Rory, who sadly passed just before the pandemic, had a wealth of knowledge in antiques, giving him and Dave a common territory to explore ... but it was the love of whisky and good food they bonded over most of all.

In another picture I can spot Suzanna Allaun's smiling face. Susz is a beautiful friend Dave kept from the time they both worked as makeup artists. She has her magic, Susz, always accepting us as we were with a wealth of kindness and knowledge. She was there for Dave in his major life moments before I came into the picture and then graciously took me and Iza into her fold too. I've learned a lot about Dave from talking to her because she has so many stories from the past working with famous faces (good and bad) and being involved in big cinematography moments. She had the patience of a saint recently going with me through five massive boxes of pictures that Dave kept from those early days. There were thousands of them, pictures that showed the makeup and detailed prosthetics for different characters in movies or on TV series.

'He was brilliant at doing this! So much talent!' she told me.

And here she is, in this picture, evidently happy for us on our wedding day.

Graham Twyford is in another picture – how Dave admired him! They became friends in school, both artists with a shared love for painting and for how art can have such a magical influence on people's lives. They went on to study together at Goldsmiths and Dave would say lovingly of Graham, 'He has the talent to build a career and put food on his family's table just by using a paintbrush. And he's become the best artist Cumbria can offer nowadays.'

Now here's a picture of the Eastons. Dr Dave and his three children, Amy, Sian and Calum, who grew up with Dave as part of the family. What memories we made with them over the years. They adopted me immediately. I think Dr Dave, who always had a camera to hand, is responsible for a fair few of the pictures in this box.

I'm glad for every one of them.

How lucky was I to have all these adventures with somebody I loved so much! How amazing it is to have had my life shaped and enriched by all these moments when my heart was so full. Full of beauty, love, connection and happiness. That is what helps. Revisiting the past via photographs is easing my journey through grief.

I haven't lost anything.

But while this trip down memory lane has turned out to be a lovely little diversion from the task at hand, I still haven't found a good enough picture of me and Dave together to give to the journalist. I give it one final rummage and ... a-ha! I land on a snap that looks easy enough to manipulate – I reckon I'll be able to crop out one of the faces.

Sorry, Simon!

Chapter Seven

Dave the Showman

Fry the onions until they're as transparent as a Geordie lass's frock!

I'll never forget the words that came down the phone line.

'Guess what, Lil?' said Dave, excitedly. 'I've had a double dip!'

He was calling me from the *Strictly Come Dancing* tanning tent where he'd just witnessed one of the show's handsome ballroom professionals, Artem Chigvintsev, having his rippling body sprayed twice for a deeper colour and Dave was impressed with what he'd seen.

'Do to me what you just did to Artem because I want to look like him,' he'd instructed the beleaguered *Strictly* spray tanner. When I saw the results of the 'double dip' for myself the next day, I couldn't help but laugh because, of course, a spray tan didn't make him look anything like Artem. He actually resembled a panda because they'd sprayed him with his glasses on.

Gosh, the *Strictly* days were a riot. You see, Dave had a naughty little gremlin who lived full-time on his shoulder, pushing him to do things that were new, daring and different, forever bringing out his mischievous side.

'Go on … do it!' it would tell him.

Not that Dave ever needed much persuading.

And so, when *Strictly* came knocking in 2013, despite never having danced a step in his life apart from the shapes he threw after a few pints of beer, it was the little gremlin who spoke to him.

Oh yes! My lovely man was 'chuffed as nuts'. Doing something like *Strictly* had been a goal of his for a long time. It was right up his street because Dave was a born performer – sometimes even putting on a show in his sleep. One night when we were in a hotel on holiday, I'd woken to Dave, butt naked, cooking in the wardrobe while still fast asleep. He was stirring pots, switching spoons, reaching for pans and talking through whatever he was preparing in great detail. I just watched and laughed and he had no recollection of any of it the next morning.

Between him and Si, I'd say Dave was the more playful. He loved the glitz and glamour, the red carpet events, and the novelty of moving in those star-studded circles never wore off.

They were both invited in 2016 to join the legendary Grand Order of Water Rats, a charitable British showbusiness fraternity made up of the great and good from the world of entertainment. You can't apply to join, you have to be proposed and seconded by existing members, and in Dave and Si's case that was Roy Wood and Rick Wakeman.

Apparently the Rats were keen to have a duo on the books as they'd not had one since Stan Laurel and Oliver Hardy.

Well Dave, tickled pink to be asked, accepted with glee. Si, on the other hand, only accepted because it brought Dave so much pleasure and later stepped back as it wasn't his type of thing. See? They didn't do *everything* together!

Even though *Strictly* was all of Dave's showbiz dreams come true, during the build-up there were definitely moments of, 'Oh my god, what have I done?!' But when it came to the crunch, Dave just went for it, refusing to allow his lack of dancing ability to hold him back. His professional partner, Karen Hauer, used to say, 'My darling, you don't have two left feet, you have *seven* left feet!' but Dave lapped up the whole experience; the sequins, Lycra and copious fake tan.

When he was launched onto the *Strictly* dancefloor on Saturday, 28 September, I was in the audience (as I would be every week) sitting alongside Iza and Sergiu, on pins with the anticipation of it all. Dave and Karen were dancing a Cha Cha Cha (of sorts) to Maroon 5's 'Moves Like Jagger', a song choice he thought showed the production team were in possession of a wicked sense of humour, and my heart was thumping out of my chest as he took to the floor dressed in a white satin sequinned shirt slashed to the navel.

As for the routine ... well, I don't think anyone had ever seen anything quite like it! Dave was jumping up and down, strutting about 'like a constipated peacock' (his words), waving his arms around, pointing manically, and at one point he dragged Karen along the floor like a sack of potatoes, which made me cry laughing. He was having such a great time and got so carried away in the moment that he finished the dance with a jubilant yell of, 'BOOM!' which definitely hadn't been part of the plan.

There was a standing ovation in the studio. Everybody was wiping away tears from the laughter, we could all see how much he was enjoying himself. Sir Bruce Forsyth, hosting what would be his final series, told Dave and Karen they were his 'favourites' (Brucie's famous *Strictly* catchphrase was the ultimate accolade) and, once she'd composed herself, new judge Darcey Bussell declared, 'Strangely, I'm in love!' Dave was ever so pleased with that one. 'Darcey's in love with me, you know,' he said later, proud as punch.

Bruno Tonioli described it as an 'insanely hilarious mess' while head judge Len Goodman said it was 'more stagger than Jagger'.

The only person who didn't like it was *Strictly*'s notoriously hard-to-impress judge Craig Revel Horwood who sat there with an icy stare, completely appalled by what he'd just witnessed on the dancefloor. He said it was 'terrifying', that Dave's gyrating had made him 'recoil in horror', and he awarded them a paltry two points for the performance, eliciting a chorus of boos from the audience.

Dave and Karen might have been up against some excellent celebrity dancers such as actress Natalie Gumede, TV presenter Susanna Reid and the model Abbey Clancy, who went on to lift the glitterball trophy, but they brought the entertainment factor in spades. Their paso doble to Meat Loaf's 'I'd Do Anything for Love' in week three and Dave's animated cape action had to be seen to be believed.

It didn't matter that he had 'seven left feet', or even what the judges thought, it was the people at home who counted and they loved watching Dave and Karen. Despite the fact that the two of them were permanently rooted to the bottom of the leaderboard, they survived week after week because the public voted them through.

Karen was lovely with Dave, although she was also strict, which he was very accepting of. He knew that she knew best and he respected her expertise and occasionally unorthodox methods. One day, exasperated with his slouchy posture and in an attempt to get him to walk with a straight spine, she tied a broom to his back. She also had some hilarious but effective techniques for helping him keep to the rhythm and would get him to chant, 'Beans on toast! Beans on toast!' as he moved through the sequence of the steps. She was so kind and patient with him and even forgave him when he managed to drop her on the floor while practising a lift.

Dave's ambition was to be able to lift Karen as effortlessly as Ben Cohen lifted his partner, Kristina Rihanoff.

'Ben, tell me how you do it,' he'd beg.

But Ben was an ex-England rugby player, built like a brick house, and there was no comparison between their two physiques.

Over the months of training, rehearsals and live shows, Dave and Karen developed a terrific relationship and she remained in our lives long after *Strictly* ended. She paid a beautiful tribute to him after he passed, calling him the partner who was closest to her heart and crediting him with teaching her not to take life too seriously. That meant a lot.

Dave never tried any of the moves he'd learned on me, though. Once he'd danced with Karen, everything else was second rate and if I ever offered to help him practise, he'd say, 'But you're not the world Mambo champion, Lil.'

Which was true, I'll give him that.

At the time of *Strictly* we owned a houseboat named Ollie, a beautiful 55-foot-long Dutch barge bought after several fun canal holidays, which we kept moored in the marina at Caversham. Ollie was more like a small apartment than a boat, with a big bedroom at the back and living space downstairs, a fully fitted kitchen, a dining table for six, two leather sofas, a fireplace and a wall-mounted TV. Proper! And the marina itself was lovely, like a floating village just off the River Thames.

Dave would stay there during the week so he and Karen could train together in London and I'd travel down from Barrow to join him every weekend. The first thing I'd do when I arrived was to change the bedsheets which were always stained bright orange from his fake tan!

Our Saturdays at the BBC studios were a hoot. After the show, the team would pile into the bar at Elstree for a few drinks and when we were unceremoniously chucked out of there at midnight, we'd carry on the party back at the Premier Inn. Somebody would order a pizza delivery and Dave and I (the naughty ones) always brought the wine. We became good friends with the rest of the group and Iza taught Abbey Clancy how to twerk, which is a brilliant claim to fame.

Don't get me wrong, it wasn't all fun and games for Dave on *Strictly*. He suffered with gout in his left foot and there was one week when it became particularly inflamed and painful. It was the same week Natalie Gumede had problems with her back and she'd already been given a bye to the next round, making it difficult, if not impossible, for the producers to grant one for Dave as well.

He went to the doctor and was given cortisol injections to see him through, but I could see on the Saturday that he was really struggling. I remember Darcey commenting, 'Dave, you need to lift the balls of your feet much better!' After the show, Dave told me, 'Balls of my feet? If she only knew the response I had in my head when she said that!'

Dave and Karen got all the way to week seven before their time was up, going out in a blaze of glory with their tango to The Proclaimers' 'I'm Gonna Be (500 Miles)' and following a dance-off with the actor Mark Benton and his partner, Iveta Lukošiūtė. He was sad that the journey was over – I was too and would miss my Saturday nights cheering him on – but the public had taken him to their hearts and the prime-time exposure on the BBC's flagship show in front of millions every week was opening doors to other opportunities.

It was around this time that Si was forced to take a year out with serious illness – an aneurysm which required brain surgery and meant a long road to recovery – and the Hairy Bikers' diary was cleared for 2014.

And so, circumstances combined to allow Dave to explore some of the offers that were coming his way and he made sure to stay busy all year while visiting Simon regularly, keeping him in the loop with everything he was up to.

Dave was already a seasoned guest TV star in his own right by this time and had appeared on *Would I Lie To You?*, *Never Mind the Buzzcocks*, and in *Countdown*'s Dictionary Corner. Throughout 2014, he racked up stints on *Room 101* and *Through the Keyhole* and that summer filmed *The Great British Sewing Bee Celebrity Special* for Children in Need, which was my favourite show on TV.

About a week before they started shooting, I gave him a crash course in sewing, showing him how to put in a zip, what an overlocker was used for and helping him put pieces of fabric together to assemble a garment. Although we nearly divorced in the process (and I feared for the health of my precious sewing machine), his ambition and enthusiasm never waned and when he casually informed the *Sewing Bee* judging panel, 'I'm now going to overlock my dress', they were bowled over. The best piece he created was a sixties-style patterned frock which ended up raising a lot of money for charity at auction.

That year he also filmed *All Star Family Fortunes* with me, Iza, Sergiu and our friend Steve who completed the Myers' team. Dave's cousin Angus was our reserve player, but his services weren't required so he remained in the green room while the rest of us were filming and ended up getting very merry with the mother of another contestant over several glasses of wine. We thought this was hysterical when we were reunited with him after the show.

We were up against *Coronation Street* star Jack P. Shepherd and his family that day and managed to beat them to reach the final where Dave and Steve were aiming to bag £10,000 for charity.

Poor Steve was doing well until he had a rabbit-in-the-headlights moment and went to pieces, dropping an almighty clanger on the question to 'name a sport without a ball'. He could have said badminton, boxing, ice hockey, darts, swimming or any number of alternatives.

'Tobogganing,' answered Steve, knowing immediately that he was going to hear the show's famous 'urgh-urgh' sound effect. He's never quite lived that down.

Nevertheless, we won the money, which we split between the Ray Armstrong Foundation and an orphanage in Romania that Dave and I had supported for a number of years, and we'd all had a fabulous day out. We went out to celebrate at Bob Bob Ricard in central London where there's a button at each table you can 'Buzz for champagne'.

And 'buzz' we did! We did some serious damage that night.

* * *

A few months after *Strictly*, Dave and Karen were booked to dance at the Variety Club charity dinner at The Savoy where there was an auction held to fundraise for a new wing at King's College Hospital. There was only one item on the list that Dave was determined to win – a 'Chanel Experience' which included tickets to the spring fashion show in Paris, a visit to the private apartment of Coco Chanel on Rue Cambon and a night in a beautiful hotel.

He knew I'd give my right arm for that and so shortly after he and Karen had performed, Dave – dressed in Lederhosen (don't ask) – turned his attention to bidding for the Chanel lot. He found himself up against Nicole Scherzinger, who seemed just as keen to bag it, but knowing how much I loved Chanel made Dave resolute and he won! He came home such a happy bunny.

The week before we left for Paris, he took me to the Chanel store in London to buy a few items – a girl can't go to a Chanel show without some Chanel. We were treated like royalty in there and given champagne and chocolate truffles and Dave sat on the sofa watching me try this and that, enjoying the whole affair with me.

I bought two jackets, a pair of boots and a bag. And that

was before we'd even got to Paris. That Chanel Experience ended up costing Dave his entire *Strictly* fee …

We made a weekend out of it, booking a second night in the same hotel and arranging to meet some friends while we were there. After visiting Coco Chanel's apartment on the Saturday morning, we had lunch and a romantic stroll through Paris before heading back to the hotel to get ready for dinner.

Dave had made a reservation at a very upmarket Italian restaurant near Place de la Concorde, even though the only table they had available was at 6.30pm, which was earlier than we'd normally eat. When we got there, we ordered some champagne and everything seemed fine until Team Chanel came in. We recognised them from the group trip to the apartment earlier in the day – there were catwalk models, PRs and stylists and the moment they sat down, the waiters completely forgot about me and Dave.

It was like we didn't exist anymore. We sat there being ignored while they fawned over the Chanel table. Dribs and drabs of food came to us at random intervals and were plonked down without any care or courtesy. The service was appalling and the meal distinctly average – certainly nothing to write home about. When we asked for the bill, it never arrived so we eventually decided to head to the till ourselves and ask again. A lady, who I assumed was the manager, maybe even the owner, made the mistake of enquiring, 'So, how was your meal?' And Dave replied.

'Well, since you ask – and I would never have mentioned it if you hadn't – we didn't have any bread on the table, your vitello tonnato was very dry, and my wife's truffle risotto had burnt oil on top. And no truffles.'

There was a couple of seconds of stunned silence as the woman's jaw dropped. And then she absolutely exploded.

'The vitello tonnato is NOT dry!' she shouted.

'Believe me, madam,' said Dave very calmly, 'I do know what I'm talking about and the vitello tonnato was definitely dry.'

'You, get out of my restaurant!'

'No, I want to pay my bill,' Dave insisted.

'Get out of my restaurant, I don't want to see you in here ever again!'

'I was only giving you a bit of feedback, I'd still like to pay for our meal.'

Bear in mind that we'd had that bottle of champers, a bottle of very good wine plus whatever the dinner was, and so the bill was a big one.

But when she told us to leave for a third time, we took the hint.

As we headed out the door, I turned to Dave and said loudly, 'Oh, darling, we must come here tomorrow night as well. It's *awfully* cheap.' That made him cry with laughter and he loved telling that story in the years to come, delivering the killer final line with relish every time.

Eating out wasn't just about the quality of the food for Dave and one of his biggest bugbears was poor service because he wanted the whole dining experience to feel elevated. There was a family holiday to LA where we went to a restaurant owned by an A-list Hollywood actress where the food was fine, but the service was so lackadaisical and slow that some of our meals arrived cold. We attempted to raise it with staff but they were just kids who didn't seem particularly bothered and it spoiled what should have been a special night out. When the bill arrived, everything was itemised by hand and at the bottom, someone had written 'tip' alongside a dash so we could fill in an amount for service.

I must point out that we always paid the gratuity and never quibbled over bills, but this time Dave was really annoyed and he wanted to let them know! He rooted around in his wallet to find every last cent owed for the bill itself and then next to 'tip' he wrote, 'Bollocks.'

* * *

A few years into the Hairy Bikers, one of the clear signs that Dave and Si were growing as entertainers and performers was the success of the live shows that they toured the length and breadth of the country with. Those tours were so special and proved to be a huge hit with audiences, with all the bedlam you'd expect from a show directed by Bob Mortimer. Neither Dave nor Si were shy about getting naked for the sake of entertainment. Especially not Dave who had no inhibitions whatsoever. At one point they came out on stage with only a bike helmet each to protect their modesty.

'May contain nuts,' was written on those helmets.

Each night would begin with the two of them talking about some of their most extraordinary experiences, all prompted by images on a big screen. After that, they'd invite somebody from the audience to come up on stage to cook with them and, naturally, the whole thing would descend into madness. I remember on the first four-month-long *Hairy Bikers' Big Night Out* tour the big finale was Dave donning a skintight silver all-in-one and dancing around the stage to Bon Jovi's 'Livin' on a Prayer' while throwing roses into the crowd.

Now, just prior to this, we'd been on a long weekend to Amsterdam where a Brit who ran an underwear shop recognised Dave on the street and asked him if he'd have a chat with his mum, who was a huge fan, on the phone. Dave would get requests like that a lot and was always quite happy to oblige. After a quick chat with the mother, this guy asked us into his store to see if there was anything we'd like to buy. That's when Dave spotted a pair of underpants that had a stuffed pouch at the front and, thinking of the tight Lycra costume he was due to wear on stage the following week, decided it would be a laugh to make a purchase.

'At least I can make my bulge a little bit bigger,' he reasoned.

Dave leaping around the stage in those chicken-fillet underpants was one of the funniest things I've ever seen. You could always rely on Mr Myers to go the extra mile.

They toured again in 2013 and this time the show required Dave to wear a red sequinned dress with a feather boa, fishnet tights and sparkly high heels. But, of course. I had to go and buy him most of the gear – talk about things you never expect to be doing for your husband, right? The only item we hadn't managed to find was the perfect pair of red heels. One day on a weekend away, I spotted some in a shop window. They were cheap, the heel was high but not too high and – best of all – they had them in a size ten. Dave tried on one of the shoes in the shop and we bought them, but on returning home we realised the box contained two shoes for the same foot!

Talk about having two left feet …

Luckily, I managed to source a pair of red Dorothy shoes from Amazon and so Dave did get to go to the ball after all.

The boys had the time of their lives doing those shows, especially enjoying the meet and greets afterwards where they got to chat to their fans on a more personal level. For all their mucking around and kiddish natures, Dave and Si were old-school pros who kept to their word, turned up and got the job done. Dave used to say, 'We might talk bollocks, but we're always on time.' He couldn't stand the thought of disappointing people and he *hated* to be late. If he'd promised to be somewhere at two o'clock, he made it his mission to be there at ten to.

In April 2010, in between dates for the first tour, Dave and I had flown to Germany for the weekend to go to a

Scorpions concert and unfortunately our flight home was cancelled due to the Icelandic ash cloud. Around 100,000 flights right across Europe were grounded during the crisis and we had no way of getting home. There were thousands of people at the airport; it was chaos and confusion for everyone and devastation on our part when we understood the implications.

Dave was beside himself, knowing they had a sell-out show in Blackpool the following night. We even investigated booking a private jet which would have cost an arm and a leg, but he would have paid it because he was so distressed about letting people down. In the end they had to cancel the show and reschedule and it took him quite a while to get over the upset. That's how much it meant to him.

The tours also turned out to be an effective barometer for what was happening in terms of the Hairy Bikers' audience. It wasn't just middle-aged men they appealed to. There were men, women and children from right across the generations and from all different backgrounds – the boys broke down barriers and had the sort of cut-through most TV stars could only dream of.

The friendship they shared on screen and on stage was exactly as it was behind the scenes in real life. They were friends for over a decade before they became TV partners and their relationship, already extremely close when I met them, only strengthened in the subsequent years. They even had matching tattoos, inked together while filming in

Argentina in 2006. I think there had probably been some drink taken, but I remember Dave calling me to say, 'Lil, what would you say about waking up in the morning with another man on your pillow?'

He'd had Che Guevara tattooed on his right upper arm, as had Si.

He joked that when I married him I also married Si, and there was more than a grain of truth in that. Indeed, many of our Valentine's Days were spent with the three of us because it just so happened that work meant Dave and Si were filming in our house around that date or there was an event in London that brought us all together.

A fan of the boys once said to me, 'It must be so much fun living with the Hairy Bikers!' I couldn't convince him that the fun I had at home was only with my husband, and definitely not as part of a threesome. When I told Dave about the exchange later, he couldn't stop laughing.

Very often people weren't able to distinguish one from the other. Dave would frequently be called Si (and vice versa) by those who approached him in the street or at events. He was always thrilled to bits about this because it meant that in the public eye, the brand was bigger than them as individuals. I stopped counting the times the two of us were eating in a restaurant and Dave would be asked, 'Where's your pal?' Sometimes they'd nod over to me and then whisper conspiratorially in Dave's ear, 'I won't tell your mate that you're out with a woman ...'

The love, affection and affinity he and Si had for each other translated onto the screen with such great effect, resonating with so many, and I know it felt quite groundbreaking given the fact that men tend to find it more difficult than women to allow themselves to be vulnerable. The public connected with them because they were completely authentic – their recipe for success was always staying true to their roots and making everything they did relatable to people right across the spectrum. They were loved by mums, dads, the young and old, bikers and foodies. Even Prince Philip was a fan.

There was a mutual respect between the boys and their audience and they always made time for the people who followed them. 'Without them, we'd be nothing,' Dave used to say. I remember he received a letter one day from a lady who very politely asked Dave if he could sign an enclosed birthday card for her husband who was sick in hospital.

'Lil,' said Dave, reading the note, 'I've got a feeling about this one ...'

Later that day, he went to the shops, bought two Hairy Bikers books (we didn't have any spare in the house that weren't stained by cooking ingredients), signed them and sent them to the lady together with the birthday card. A couple of weeks later we received another letter from the same lady who told us Dave's gesture had brightened her husband's final days and that the day before he passed, he'd used one of the books to write down his legacy wishes for his unborn grandson.

Dave and Me

Dave was deeply moved by that and there are many other examples of exchanges just like it that showed the special connection the boys shared with their viewers. Throughout the years they remained consistent and never tried to be something they were not. They wouldn't have known how.

A key element to their magic formula was that they only ever *offered* their knowledge, they never tried to teach. The best teachers are always the ones who make learning fun and that's what Dave and Si did – if you do what you love, others will see that and receive it.

In business and in friendship they knew they could wholly rely on each other and that is rare. Dave and Si would finish each other's sentences, knowing intuitively what the other was about to say about a recipe or a method of cooking. The freedom they enjoyed in the kitchen was because neither had any of the constraints of formal training. Both had learned to cook out of necessity and their love of food was born from hardship.

Dave would even have conversations with Si in his sleep – deep discussions about recipes and ingredients.

'No, no, that's not right, Kingy. Add a bit of this in, try that!'

One night, he was having one of these talks and becoming quite animated despite being fast asleep and I just put my hand on him to try to calm it down a little.

'Don't touch my bum, Kingy!' he said, not even waking.

Between series, the two of them would take off for boys' weekends – getting sloshed in an ice bar in Iceland or enjoying the fine dining in Niklas Ekstedt's restaurant in Stockholm. These guys sure knew how to have fun together. I feel incredibly lucky to have had a front-row seat as this beautiful friendship developed into a wonderful on-screen partnership, one which brought happiness to so many.

They really were a team in every sense.

* * *

I must tell you about the time Dave and I nearly got arrested in Egypt. In October 2014, he was filming there for an episode of the BBC series *A Cook Abroad*.

For context, this was a period when the country was on high alert after the Islamic State had taken four Western aid workers hostage in Syria. Dave and the team were given a military escort the whole time they were filming there. On the day they were wrapping the episode, I flew to meet him in the city of Luxor where he had arranged for someone to pick me up from the airport and bring me to the hotel. It was a massive complex with around 1,000 rooms, but given the political situation, today it was deserted. On the surrounding streets there was barbed wire erected everywhere with a strong military presence and it all amounted to a very eerie atmosphere.

I was shown to the room and Dave arrived shortly after me, covered in sand, having been filming with the Nubians, an ethnic group who live in the Nile Valley. After a quick kiss and a 'hello, darling', he jumped straight in the shower.

He'd left his bags in the hotel lobby to be put through the X-ray machine, which was a requirement in any building at that point.

The phone in our room rang.

'Mr Myers, come to the reception immediately, this is an emergency,' said the voice on the other end of the line. I explained that my husband was in the shower and would come down as soon as he was dressed.

'No, ma'am. You must come to the reception, NOW.'

This sounded deadly serious. I was scared, wondering what on earth was happening that required such urgency. I took the lift down to the lobby where I was escorted into a room with lots of screens and six people stood with guns around Dave's travel bag, which was on a table right in the middle.

'Madam, is this your husband's suitcase?'

I nodded. The officer pointed to a screen on the wall.

'If you look at the X-ray image you will see the shape of a gun. Your husband has a gun in his suitcase. Please open it now.'

All eyes were trained on me and they turned their guns in my direction as I stepped towards the bag. What had my man done? Many things flashed through my mind ... could he have bought a replica gun as a giggle? Oh god. We were both going to be thrown into an Egyptian prison to rot because of some stupid joke he'd had somewhere on the road.

I carefully opened the suitcase, convinced by this point that I was about to see a gun. There, sitting on top of Dave's clothes, was a brown paper package. Everyone in the room was focused on me.

This was very bad.

My hands were shaking as I started to unwrap the offending item, cursing Dave in my head for being so idiotic, only to reveal … a 30-centimetre-high model of an Egyptian deity with a gigantic penis sticking out at a right angle.

And yes, on the X-ray it looked very much like a gun.

The officers looked at me and these big guys with their lethal weapons all started to laugh. I could feel my face redden.

'Ma'am,' said the man in charge, 'it looks like your husband wanted to surprise you.'

'I'll give him a surprise now when I see him!' I replied.

I marched back to the room thinking, 'I'm going to get you, Mr Myers!'

It turned out that Dave, who was still in the shower and had missed all this commotion, had spotted this statue in a shop and thought it would make an amusing present for Si. When I told him what had happened, both of us fell about laughing. Honestly, this is the sort of absurdity that could only have happened to Dave Myers.

As if life couldn't get more comical, not long after returning from Egypt, Dave took on what promised to be his maddest challenge yet and signed up for his panto debut. I'll be honest, when I saw my first pantomime years ago, it screwed with my head. We don't have anything like an equivalent in Romania and the entire thing with all its innuendo and twisted fairy tales blew my mind. I've been in the UK for 20 years and I still think it's completely bonkers.

Dave was given the role of Baron Hardup in Reading's Hexagon Theatre production of *Cinderella*. We worked together on it because I was hired to be part of the costume team and this was how Dave's now-famous twirly moustache came into being. We were preparing for a photocall and Dave was trying out his Baron's costume. We'd given him these painted red, rosy cheeks and I suggested he twiddled with his tache a little, maybe curling it up at each end for an added flourish.

Well, he loved it.

He loved it so much that after the panto run had finished, he decided to keep it, which I was very pleased about because it suited him so well. It added to his smiley face and reflected his personality and joy – it soon became hard to imagine him without it. The tache became Dave's new obsession. The number of products he had for keeping it groomed and in place was borderline ridiculous. He had these tiny combs that he'd keep in his pocket so he could give it a little flick if it ever started to droop. And what a drama it would be in the morning if he couldn't locate a comb.

While working on the panto, we lived on board Ollie and became ensconced in the community on the marina. We felt at home there. All the boats were decorated with thousands of twinkly lights, smoke coming out of their little chimneys, and the vibes were so cosy and welcoming.

We were working with actors from all different areas of the country and since many did not have plans for New Year's Eve, obviously we had to throw a big party. Dave invited everyone to the boat and not having time to cook, what with doing two shows a day, we shopped at Costco and bought various semi-prepared foods and plenty of drinks.

We had biscuits, prawn cocktails and a decorated fillet of salmon – we even found a wedge of truffle cheese that smelled divine. When our guests arrived, we took them all to the pub for a pint and an eighties disco before heading back to the boat for champagne, food and more dancing.

I was having such a good time that I hadn't noticed quite a few items of food disappearing from the table, but the next morning we kept getting a waft of something pungent. After sniffing high and low, we figured out that Snowy, our Westie, was trumping out truffle-scented farts. And that's when we realised that we'd not seen hide nor hair of that huge great lump of cheese the night before. Amid all the merriment, Snowy must have carried out a sneaky raid on the table and, although I doubted he'd been able to eat the whole lot, we could only find a few chewed-up pieces hidden under the sofa some days later. From that day to the day we lost him six years later, he was known by all our friends as the truffle-farting dog. Bless little Snowy.

We'd rung in 2015 with our panto family, full of hope for the year ahead. Si's health had vastly improved and the boys started making plans to work together again. They took to the road to film *The Hairy Bikers' Pubs That Built Britain* and Dave was happy as Larry to be back on the bike with his best mate.

And ticking away in the background was another dream he was about to make a reality.

The Hat

23 October 2024

I'm sitting with a cup of coffee in the best spot in the house. It's a round sofa in the large bay window of the dining room, positioned for unspoiled views of the parkland outside. I can see the gentle ripples on the lake and a few geese waddling on the well-manicured lawn.

There's not a soul around.

On one corner of the sofa's backrest hangs a straw hat.

Dave's holiday hat.

It travelled the globe with us (and the Bikers) and it's like he's right here next to me as I quietly sip my coffee and watch the world outside. Travel was such a big part of our life together – Dave had wanderlust in his bones and holidays were always adventurous, opportunities to explore new cultures, people and, of course, food.

The first big holiday we had as a family was to Jamaica in 2009 shortly after the boys had filmed *The Hairy Bikers: Mums Know Best*. One of the contributors to the series was a wonderful Jamaican mum called Connie who had told Dave all about the Caribbean island's bold, flavoursome food, which is steeped in tradition and full of slow-cooked jerk chicken goodness. That was more than enough to sell it to Mr Myers. I remember him coming back from filming that episode saying, 'Right, we have to go to Jamaica.' Which is exactly what we did.

We paid a fortune for what was an amazing trip, the first time we'd been able to afford a holiday quite like that.

After filming in wondrous places around the world, Dave always wanted to take my hand and show me his playgrounds. We'd go to Bruges to drink beer with Bertie (a professor of beer!), to Seoul and the Gangnam district, to Tokyo where we ate in the same small street-food places with the 'salarymen' behind the Shibuya Crossing. From Mumbai to Marrakech, so many memories experienced together – now my constellation of glimmers.

Dave would always conduct meticulous research before booking to make sure wherever we were going would be the best. He'd do all the necessary homework on the local restaurant options, trawling the Tripadvisor reviews and cross-referencing with other platforms to come up with a list of gems to venture to. His methods were thorough but not always foolproof, and there were times when we'd arrive somewhere and he'd refuse to set foot over the threshold. If, for instance, there were photographs of the food on the door, that was a big no-no for him and he'd usher us away to find an alternative place to eat, me hobbling on my high heels and cursing myself for not wearing flats.

In December 2015, while en route from LA to Las Vegas, we stopped off in Big Bear Lake for a couple of nights where Dave had booked us into the most outlandish of lodgings called Castle Wood Cottages. The place was a bit like stepping into a fairy tale – Sergiu's room was a cave with rock walls, stalagmites and crystals, while Iza's was forest themed with trees and live woodland animals. Dave and I were in an enchanted castle with a bedroom up in a tower, a spiral staircase and an actual moat flowing through the middle of the space. Places like this always put a grin on Dave's face, playing right into his childlike nature.

We were there for two nights, one of which was my birthday, and Dave did his usual online investigation to find us a decent place to eat. The top-rated eatery on Tripadvisor was closed so he settled on the second one and we arrived with high hopes. We were greeted by a tall, handsome gent who took us to our seats and informed us that there were no menus.

'Here,' he said, 'we feed you.'

OK, we replied, slightly dubious but happy to go along with this novel way of doing things. We explained that Iza was vegetarian ('Don't worry, we will feed you all!'), and Dave added that it was my birthday so could we have a bottle of champagne to celebrate? 'Ohhh, I've got something better than that!' replied our man, awfully pleased with himself. He returned to our table – and I promise this is true – with a bottle of Lambrusco. The kind you can buy in Tesco for £1.50.

But this guy was so proud of his restaurant. Even the Wi-Fi password was 'delicious'. Anyway, the first course arrived. It was a pineapple quarter with the flesh scooped and diced and with some sort of red sauce on top. We looked at it and then at each other, eyebrows decidedly raised. And then we tasted it and realised the red sauce was tomato ketchup. We couldn't decide if someone was having a laugh at our expense.

The second course was even worse. Chopped up pieces of boiled chicken and some very stiff spaghetti which tasted like it had been cooked two days before. Iza's veggie substitute for the chicken was yet more pineapple on top of the same spaghetti.

You may wonder why we didn't get up and leave, but we were finding the experience so flipping funny that we had to stay and see it through. The staff were so elated with what they were serving up and the reviews were all pretty good so at one point we started to wonder if *we* were the problem! Perhaps it was a case of American tastes and expectations being wildly different to our own. Whatever it was, the meal was worth every dollar for the entertainment value we had from the whole experience.

Of all the beautiful places we visited together I'd say Thailand was our favourite. It was the kindness and friendliness of the Thai people that made it so unique – you'd only need to catch someone's eye to get a huge, sunny smile in return.

We first went there in December 2012, and I remember the excitement and anticipation when Dave, feeling flush, booked business-class flights for all of us. This was a first for me and the kids and it took a huge chunk of our budget, but Dave said, 'This is too much of an occasion not to experience something like this together. I want to see Sergiu and Iza's faces when we turn left on the plane and get to their seats!' Well, their faces were indeed a picture when we boarded.

'Mum, Dave, look at this, I can turn my seat into a bed!' squealed Iza, getting a taste of how the other half lived. They lapped up the luxury, feasting on the food which was a distinct cut above what we were used to in economy.

'Now look, kids,' said Dave, 'don't get used to this because it's a treat and it's not going to happen very often ...'

We spent Christmas in Bangkok in a hotel right on the Chao Phraya River. After that we moved on to the island of Koh Samui with its palm trees, crystal waters and white sandy beaches and where we rented scooters, dodging the tourist traps to eat where the locals did. Dave was always in search of the most authentic food. 'We go where the locals go, because that is where the real food is,' he'd say. The respect he had for local people wherever his travels took him always transpired in his stories.

The New Year's Eve moon party on Bophut Beach was something else. Thousands of people gathered on the sand, there were acrobats with fire torches, plastic buckets filled with deliciously sugary cocktails, music, dancing, laughing gas and cigars. What a phenomenal atmosphere with people from all over the world. We were so carried away with it all that we forgot we had our mobiles in our pockets as we ran into the sea to join a communal moon dance.

Back at the hotel in the early hours of the morning, something happened that we laughed about for years. Because the sand had managed to find a way into every crevasse, Dave went straight into the shower, but thanks to a few too many of the strong cocktails, he slipped and fell, hitting his arm quite badly on the way down. While I was trying to help him up, there was an urgent knock at the door and my daughter shouting, 'Mum, come quickly!'

Sergiu, who was staying with Iza in the adjacent room, had somehow fallen asleep in their bathtub fully clothed. So here we were, Iza and I, trying to lift two substantially heavy, worse-for-wear males, one off the floor and one out of a bathtub to put them to bed.

Dave kept saying he'd broken his arm, although he stubbornly refused to go to the hospital and eventually passed out in a happy state of drunkenness. In the morning neither he nor Sergiu could remember much at all and so me and Iza gladly filled in the blanks. No arms had been broken, thank goodness, but the same couldn't be said for our phones. They'd been completely submerged in the sea and were very dead and no amount of rice drying could revive them. Worth it, though!

Such carefree, blessed and unforgettable family times.

Gosh, this hat has just taken me on quite the journey ... Teddy has come to join me (and the hat), snuggling down on the floor by my feet. Everything is still and silent, but not inside my head where my thoughts are rampant. I can now feel Dave's presence so strongly that it's almost as if his lips are touching my coffee cup.

Oh, my darling. You must have been so scared and felt so alone in all the physical torment you went through. I was there for you every second of the day and night, but this dreadful illness separated us no matter how close our hearts were. I remember the look on your face each morning when I'd open my eyes and catch you staring at me. It was clear you were not well, but you forced a smile to make me feel better, and I want you to know that not once in those moments did I abandon hope that things could turn around and become different for us. If only hope could cure, I would have had enough to cure you and the rest of the world.

My coffee tastes salty now that I'm back to this reality without you, here in this beautiful house you chose for us.

I reach out and stroke the hat.

I couldn't be more grateful to have walked alongside you for the past 20 years, and now I'm sitting in the silence of life continuing without you. Empty of you. But you are the presence that is never an absence.

Chapter Eight

French Dream

That marinade will stick to the chicken like a Jack Russell hanging on to the vicar's trousers!

Our French adventure began after a family boating holiday had ended in disaster.

It was Easter 2014 and we'd taken our Dutch barge Ollie out for a week on the Thames with the kids, the weather forecast firmly on our side as we set off. On the first night we stopped near the village of Sonning where Uri Geller had a 25 metre long mooring spot which boaters could use as long as they popped ten pounds through a mailbox bearing the message, 'I'm watching you, put a tenner through.'

Ha! Dave loved this funny touch from Mr Geller.

All was going well until the following evening when we reached our second stop a little bit further down the river at Henley and noticed something wasn't right with Ollie. He'd started to take in water through the gland – not that any of us novices knew what a 'gland' in a boat was ...

turns out, it's pretty essential. And it put a stop to our trip up the Thames.

Dave was determined we were still going to have a holiday, so we put Ollie into a local yard for repairs and got a lift back to our car at the marina at Caversham. We organised for Snowy to go to the kennels for a few days and all jumped in the car to head across the Channel to spend a long Easter weekend in France.

We stopped in Lisieux, a small town two hours south of Calais and checked into a hotel where we could walk to the cathedral for the Easter Sunday service. Within minutes of arriving in this pretty little place, we'd fallen in love with it. It was the easiness of it all, the green produce in the groceries, the patisseries, the baguettes, the charm of the cafés, the restaurants run by *les mamans* of *la famille*. The unmistakable French *je ne sais quoi*.

It made Dave and I start dreaming about getting a place of our own, not necessarily here but somewhere in rural France, which could be a project – somewhere to spend the summer months and possibly move to permanently when we retired. And once Dave Myers had an idea in his head, he would move heaven and earth to make it a reality.

Our love affair with France had really begun several years before with our trips to Nîmes in the south and the hotel Jardins Secrets, with its opulent curtains and canopied four-poster beds. Dave and I adored it there. So much so that in 2017 when the boys were in Nîmes filming *Hairy Bikers'*

Mediterranean Adventure (probably my favourite series because Dave and Si both looked so healthy and sunkissed and, in my opinion, it featured some of the best food they ever did) the director Francois Gandalfi called me to ask if I'd like to come out as a surprise.

Well, of course I would!

I think Francois had been tipped off by Si that they were in one of our favourite places and so as they were finishing off filming in the central square, I quietly stepped into shot and said, 'Hello, darling …' Dave couldn't believe it, but he was over the moon which was a relief because that man did not usually like surprises. 'There goes my pizza!' he joked because all the crew were going out to a restaurant that night and I'd scuppered his plans.

But back to 2014 when, just a couple of months after resolving to put down some roots in France, we took off on Dave's new Kawasaki bike (or the 'quickest fuckie', as he liked to call it) to scour the northwest of the country in pursuit of the perfect home. We'd each packed a pannier of items and planned to be away for a month, focusing our search around the Normandy and Brittany regions, thinking the close proximity and easy access to the Channel crossing options should be a priority. A little crash pad was what we had in mind, a compact apartment or small dwelling in the countryside. But the thing is, there were never any half-measures with Mr Myers. Whatever he was doing, it had to be with bells and whistles and so our initial, more modest plans were quickly ditched.

'Too small, won't fit a good bed.'

'Nah, it hasn't got parking space.'

'Too rural, too far away from any shops – what would we do if we wanted a baguette?'

All these, and many more, were the reasons we found – or, to be more accurate, the reasons *he* found – against the first raft of properties the estate agent showed us round.

To be fair to Dave, some of the points he raised were valid. Take the word 'rural', for instance. Rural in France means really and truly remote, completely off the beaten track and with not much in the way of neighbours or local community. We wanted somewhere that had a little bit of life and personality. We didn't want total isolation.

I'm not sure if our list of demands was getting longer, or if we were slowly excluding what would not work for us, but what did become clear was that Dave's idea of a 'crash pad' was not what we'd originally talked about. After hearing no after no from us, the under-pressure agent had one last property on her list. It was a *Maison de Maître* in Mayenne, part of the Pays de la Loire region and further south than we'd anticipated going.

When we got there, I saw Dave's eyes brighten. This was followed by a loud sigh of approval when he saw the gardens, which were quite spectacular. The top half of the space was ornamental with shrubs and hedges trimmed into the shape of hearts around a central fountain. There was a swimming pool and then a potager, or vegetable garden, which I think is what sold the place to Dave as he recognised the potential for a new venture, despite not having much experience with growing his own veg.

Having been brought up in a place with a garden and lots of open space, this was also a lovely feature for me, but if I'm completely honest it was the pool that did the trick as far as I was concerned. We were both melting from the heat in our full biking gear and the glistening water looked so appealing. I just wanted to discard the leathers and jump straight in! That swimming pool would turn out to be a source of huge fun in the years to come, but also of deep frustration when it started to leak and needed the liner changed at huge expense. It was a massive job, and because the cheap solution was never an option for Dave, the liner we put in as a replacement was the same kind they use in Olympic swimming pools.

But gosh, this house was utterly charming.

An old wisteria vine climbed the south aspect of the building, painting the wall in shades of purple and green. There was an outdoor space with an open kitchen full of possibilities (I could picture Dave cooking up a storm there) as well as a *pigeonnier*, which is a little tower dating from the Medieval age when French families raised pigeons as a source of meat. Today, we were reliably informed, it was home to a family of white owls.

The people who were selling were old money; the man had been a figure of authority in his active life and had decorated the house in a Napoleonic style to reflect their status, with hand-painted silk panels in the living room and patterned tapestry on the bedroom walls. A narrow spiral staircase was central to the property, finished with a cupola at the top which was painted with green vines and beautiful birds. The top floor was used as a playroom and Dave immediately started dreaming of creating a man cave with a train set installation, sofas, books and a TV.

The whole place was deliciously quirky and so different to anything we'd seen before. It was also triple the budget. For me, that meant there was a lot to consider but Dave's mind was made up. He wanted this house.

We returned to the UK and he had to head off for a few weeks with a busy filming schedule, but every phone call home would begin with the same question.

'Have you bought me the house?'

Dave always left the finances and the signing of large cheques to me because it made him giggle knowing how alien it was for me to deal with that amount of cash. It also meant he avoided the pain of actually seeing the money fritter away.

'We both grew up piss poor,' he'd say with a big grin, 'but you as a Romanian immigrant paying all this money takes the mick! Go on, girl, you sign that!'

By February 2015 the house was ours and this was where the fun really began. We bought a big Luton van and would go off to antique auctions in Britain or *dépôt-ventes* in France, picking up beautiful pieces of furniture, paintings and clocks for our new home. My level of French is quite good – I understand and can hold a conversation – but watching Dave attempt the language was side-splitting. He had no grasp of it much beyond *bonjour* and *merci*, but that didn't put him off engaging in arduous discussions with market stall-holders, shop assistants and our new neighbours. He'd invent words and use expressive hand gestures to somehow make himself understood.

The kids went shopping for a mattress with him once and witnessed him trying to communicate this to the assistant.

'*Monsieur, j'achète le* boing-boing?'

'*Le* boing-boing' worked and Dave came home with a new *matelas*.

Another time when the house had a small infestation of mice, he went out to buy traps.

'*Madam?*' he said to the lady in the shop. 'Um … *souris?*' He pulled a finger across his throat in a slitting motion. She understood – he came back with mouse traps!

I remember once we drove past a sign that said, '*Don de Sang*' and Dave got very excited about the possibility of a new Chinese restaurant opening in the neighbourhood. Until I told him it was actually a poster about blood donation.

Our village, Fougerolles-du-Plessis, was an idyllic place with a big church right in the centre surrounded by a square. There was a patisserie, which was impossible to resist thanks to the enticing smell of fresh baguettes and croissants every morning, a bar called GiGi's, a lovely little restaurant called Le Lion D'Or that only did lunches – 12 euro for three courses and a drink – and a town hall. Just a short walk away we had a bank, supermarket, pharmacy and a GP practice.

We based ourselves there from March to September and made many friends, French and British, in the local community. We also had a constant stream of visitors from back home because the house was the perfect space for entertaining. During one particularly raucous party we had about 50 people in the garden and one of our friends (whose identity I'll protect) woke up naked in a bush at four in the morning. Such fun nights that went on long into the early hours and usually ended up with everyone dive-bombing into the pool.

The one thing Dave wasn't happy about was the kitchen with its ancient cooking range which was impossible to bake in. As there were no other practical options – none that were good enough to pass Dave's high standards anyway – we hired a company from Kent to renovate the kitchen while, true to form, he was away filming.

It was yours truly who oversaw the work and in 2019 Dave came home to a spanking new, achingly modern kitchen with Miele appliances, a gleaming black-and-gold marble work surface (which he wasn't too sure about at first but grew to love) and a wine cooler that made him extremely happy.

The house had a wine cellar, hidden beneath the staircase and fitted with shelves that we kept well stocked. A wine trader called Emmanuel would knock at the door twice a year and take our order for anything he had on his list, which was the same every time he called. He'd bring samples with him and sit down at our kitchen table sipping a cup of coffee veeeerrrry slowly. Emmanuel spoke no word of English, but he and Dave would be engrossed in conversations nonetheless – sometimes I translated, other times I just left them to it because to listen to them chatter away was my entertainment.

Our life in France was everything we'd imagined when we'd first started dreaming. The highlight of Dave's week were Saturday mornings when we went to the market for fresh food. There was a good one only 20 minutes away in Fougères but the one he liked the most was a 40-mile drive to Rennes. Now, this place was awesome and vast – you could find anything and everything and Dave was on cloud nine whenever we went. He would touch and smell the herbs, running like an excited schoolboy from one stall to another, admiring the colour of the vegetables, enthralled by the freshness of the produce, picking up a lettuce to show me how wonderful it was. He'd weigh the tomatoes in his hands, dash between the fish stands to choose the best lobsters, detailing to me how he planned to cook them and asking questions of the traders in his broken French.

One particular Saturday, he'd bought a fabulous crystal platter featuring a lobster decoration at a *brocante* and as a man who always aimed for perfection, he said this new serving plate deserved the perfect lobster. That evening we had one of the best salads I've ever tasted made with two lobsters Dave had so carefully selected. As he always said,

'Good food and drinks have to be shared to be fully valued,' and so we invited a few friends around our outdoor table to indulge in the feast with some French vino and Debussy's *'Clair de lune'* in the background. Dave was a wizard when it came to creating beautiful and meaningful moments.

One time when he returned from filming in the Baltics, he brought home a big tin of caviar and made dozens of blinis, topped with sour cream mixed with a bunch of dill from the garden. We ate them with our favourite white wine Condrieu and watched the setting sun by candlelight, Chopin playing softly. It's hard to imagine anything more blissful ...

On rainy days in France, Dave would work on his model railway train in the attic, Project Man Cave now complete. He'd have David Bowie blasting, although not loud enough to drown out the occasional yelp of frustration if the building work wasn't quite going to plan. As ambitious as ever, he wanted to create a landscape on three levels with a train station, tunnels and bridges, villages on hills and trees with tiny little apples painted in red. He even bought miniature cabbages and carrots to 'plant' in his garden. Once the model railway was finished, Dave planned to create a 'Channel Tunnel' through the wall and then continue on the other side into the next room with a French version. When I say he didn't do things by half, this is exactly what I mean!

It was a labour of love and a constant work in progress. One he never got to complete.

* * *

I loved my French garden and worked hard to maintain the exquisitely coiffed hedges, to plant the vegetables in spring and nurture them until they offered us fresh food to enjoy. Dave was ecstatic to be able to take a little basket and 'go shopping' in his own back garden.

He googled how to grow potatoes and beans and invested in all sorts of gardening devices that I could never use and neither could he.

He once bought me a manual rotavator 'just to help you turn the beds in spring'. Try as we might, this thing only scraped the surface of the soil, so that was no good. Another day he came home with a 'muncher' that was supposed to shred the branches I'd trimmed from the shrubs and bushes. It worked for an hour before giving up the ghost altogether.

One year he decided that he wanted a greenhouse and the two of us planted vines of tomatoes, green peppers, chilli plants and pak choi – not exactly a common green to plant, but Dave was always trying something different. He experienced such joy at being able to pick the juicy red cherry tomatoes off the vines in his own greenhouse and the green beans he'd planted months before! I loved seeing him take to gardening in his energetic way, kitted out in dungarees and wellies, soil caked on his face, singing while digging his potatoes. He certainly brought the Myers brand of magic to the garden.

He also discovered another new passion while we were in France. Horse racing. It had all started with our friend Steve from the Isle of Man, who was building a family home in a

French village about 60 miles away from us where everyone was involved with horses. He'd introduced us to this exciting new world and it wasn't long before Dave was hooked. He loved the race Sundays we attended, with the horse parades and the ooohs and ahhhs from the crowd as these magnificent beasts galloped along the course.

As Dave's 60th birthday approached in 2017, I was completely stumped over what on earth to give him as a present. What do you buy a man who has almost everything?

Which is how I landed on the idea of buying him a racehorse.

I had no clue where to start, so asked Steve to help me and he enlisted a local horse trainer to join the search. About five months later, on the day of Dave's birthday, we got a call from the trainer to say that he'd found The One. This horse, Lightoller, ticked all the boxes and, at two years old, would give us a few decent racing years. Dave and I were in Mallorca celebrating his birthday with friends, so I printed a picture of the horse, putting it in an envelope along with the registration papers and a birthday card.

Dave was euphoric! I think it was his favourite present anyone had ever given him. I'd also enclosed in the envelope Lightoller's colours, which had already been assigned by the French horse racing authority and were striped grey and dusty pink.

'Exactly the colours of Christian Dior,' as Dave loved explaining to everybody.

Dave and Me

We had tremendous fun with that little horse. And Tollie, as we called him, turned out to be a very good investment – in the three years we owned him, he earned a small fortune. Racing life in France is completely different to that in Britain – it's less of a spectacle and there are no posh hats and no swanning about. It's a lot more rough and ready and inclusive. Everybody pays six euro to get in, you eat burgers, have a beer, kids and dogs run about, and it's a cheap and cheerful family day out.

On the days we attended we'd wear our owners' badges and could go to the stables where the horses were being prepared for the race. It was breathtaking to see the care they were handled with and, although in the past I'd always felt a twinge of pity for racehorses, they appeared to be very happy doing what they did.

We'd then go to the owners' enclosure to watch Tollie come out for the parade before the jockey popped in for some last-minute advice from the trainer about how to tackle the race ahead. We'd watch the jockey mount and trot over to the start which is when we'd quickly run to put a bet on our favourite. There's a whole science behind the art of placing a good bet – Steve had it mastered and Dave and I learned the ropes.

After that, we'd find a good seat, feeling the excitement building as the crowd came alive. The surge of exhilaration we all experienced if Tollie won a place on the podium was like nothing else. Dave and Steve would be hugging and

laughing and the day would always finish with a boozy, cele-
bratory lunch.

Every pub in France has screens showing races from the
courses across the country, so on the days Tollie was running
but we couldn't attend, Dave would run across the road from
our house to GiGi's bar, usually covered in soil and still in his
gardening gear, to watch it there.

'*Mon cheval! Mon cheval!*' he'd shout, pointing at the
screen. He became very popular in GiGi's because whenever
Tollie won, he'd buy everyone there a beer. It didn't matter
who they were or if he knew them, everyone would get a
drink. The locals were delighted to have a racehorse owner
living in the village, even more so when Dave passed on a
tip and they'd all place their bets accordingly. Although he
wasn't exactly flavour of the month on the odd occasion
when his tip turned out to be duff information and they lost
their three-euro investment ...

Dave had certainly caught the racing bug. So much so
that he decided to plough Tollie's winnings into buying
another two horses. Unfortunately, they turned out to be
donkeys who didn't do anything except sprain their ankles
and refuse to run. The first one was called Light Heart and
was a cast-off from Sheik Maktoum's stables, a fact that got
Dave's shoulder gremlin going enough for him to buy it.
He cost triple the amount of money I'd paid for Tollie and
gave us a grand total of two races before turning his nose
up at everything else. Light Heart, it seemed, was far more

interested in checking out the female horses than exerting himself by racing.

Then came a little yearling, who we named Dave the Great to everyone's amusement. Only he wasn't really that 'great' and never even made it to a start line. All the money we'd made on Tollie was gobbled up by Light Heart and Dave the (not so) Great and their upkeep.

Then came the pandemic so we couldn't get to France and we reached a point where we had to look at cutting our losses. We gave Light Heart to a friend who had a bit of land with other horses and Dave the Great went to our friend Steve. Poor Tollie, who had worked so hard and paid for everything else, was retired to a racehorse sanctuary and very well looked after.

All good things, as they say ... It had been fun while it lasted.

* * *

Maybe it was too good to be true.

In the summer evenings after dinner, we'd take our glasses of wine into the garden, enjoying the tranquillity and the beauty of this heavenly place we'd created together. But can anything really stay that perfect forever?

The Brexit vote of June 2016 had been loitering in the background for most of the time we'd been in France and the deal that was eventually signed in January 2020 was crushing. It curtailed the number of days Dave was allowed to be there while still running the businesses in the UK he'd taken years to build up. He wasn't a man who liked limitations and he detested being restricted in this way. The house and garden needed regular upkeep and we were now unable to be there to give them the love and attention they required.

Then came the pandemic.

Then illness.

Three catastrophes that combined to burst our bubble and shatter our dreams. Eventually, there really wasn't much choice but to sell that wonderful house in France and I would say goodbye to it the same week I buried Dave.

I took with me only memories and left behind a piece of my heart.

The Matches

2 November 2024

Some days my thoughts are so free-flowing that I feel an urge to put pen to paper and the words seem to pour onto the page. Writing brings relief and clarity as well as comfort ... if I continue to talk and write about him, so he lives on.

Today is one of those days, so I'm here at my desk to get some of it down. I'm aware that our memories are fluid and malleable, changing over time as they filter through our minds. A well-known coach, Melissa Tiers, has spoken a lot about memory consolidation and she describes the process as being similar to a Word document. Every time you open the document to edit the text, the previous version is gone forever – that's also how we access and modify our memories. Each time we retrieve them, they become a little more distorted.

I don't want my recollections of Dave to be reshaped or clouded ... I want to preserve them in their purest form so they remain as vivid as the day we lived them. And there are connections to him in every part of this house – little reminders with huge significance that spark memories of days when life was bright and shiny.

Take this box of matches on my desk, for instance. They're not just any old matches, you see. This is a limited-edition souvenir box from the 2018 Cornbury Music Festival in Oxfordshire where Dave and Si hosted a wood-fired pop-up restaurant. On one side of the colourfully designed box is that year's line-up (Alanis Morissette, UB40, Squeeze and Deacon Blue, among others) and on the other is a mini poster for the Hairy Bikers' Festival Feast. The boys performed at this event for a couple of years running and it was always an enjoyable weekend despite the long shift for Dave and Si, who were cooking in the tent from early morning until late at night.

This year was especially fun because Si's band Little Moscow were playing a set on one of the smaller stages, so after the final Festival Feast meal was served, we all went along to watch the gig where there was a fair amount of beer sunk. Dave being Dave, he was up for a party and I left him happily dancing in a field with friends at about midnight when I headed back to our Airstream caravan on the other side of the huge estate.

I went to sleep as soon as my head hit the pillow, but I didn't stay sleeping for long. At about two in the morning, I was woken by the noise of a vehicle pulling up outside. Bleary-eyed, I peered through the curtains to see my man climbing out of an ambulance. What on earth had happened?!

Dave and Me

It turned out that Dave had got hopelessly lost on his way back to our accommodation – it was dark, he'd had a few pints and couldn't for the life of him find where we were staying. In his confusion, he'd wandered into the campsite area and accidentally stumbled onto someone's tent from which a very angry bloke had emerged, ready to fight whoever had woken him up ... until he recognised Dave and immediately softened.

The guy called over to the site security guard and asked if they could help this hapless Hairy Biker get back to where he was staying.

'Where's your accommodation, Dave?' asked the guard.

'Um, it's like a caravan ... I'm not sure where it is. I don't know where I live!'

From Dave's vague description, the security and First Aid teams tried to figure out where our Airstream was and offered to drive him back. Hence the ambulance. They drove him all over the site trying to jog his memory before he spotted somewhere familiar and woke me from my slumber. He couldn't stop giggling and I couldn't be mad at him.

Mr Myers, you could charm your way out of anything ...

When I find items like this box of matches and they take me on a trip to the past, the memories triggered aren't painful now – I make a point of saving them into my bank of happy times, separate from the memories of when Dave was ill, because that wasn't him.

We have two choices over how we look back. We can feel awful that the happy moments have gone, or we can see them as something beautiful, feel grateful that they happened at all and allow them to bring us consolation.

I choose the latter.

Just recently, the Buddhist parable of the two arrows came to my attention and it really spoke to me. When a person is struck by an arrow – a terrible event – it is impossible to avoid. This could be the death of a loved one, a job loss that puts us in a financially precarious situation, a relationship struggle or a critical decision that turns out to be catastrophic. We will all encounter chaos like this – pain, personal challenges and complexities that threaten to derail us. And when that arrow hits, my god, it hurts like hell.

The second arrow represents our response to the first: it's the manner in which we choose to react. If we attach ourselves to the pain of the first arrow and wallow in it, continuing to think all the negative thoughts it brought about, then we send a second arrow hurtling straight into our open wound.

In other words, it's not what happens to us but the way we react to it that dictates the depth of our pain. Whether we are hit twice can be entirely within our control. It's not about denying our feelings. But by taking a moment to breathe and becoming aware of our emotional response, we can make a choice about how to proceed.

I don't want the tragedy of losing Dave to define me or dictate my narrative and I won't allow it to. I will write the next chapter of my life learning from the past, not being limited by it and by feeling joy remembering the good times just as they happened.

My plan is to use all of that to strengthen my steps on the path I'm paving for myself.

Chapter Nine

Pandemic

That's hotter than a welder's clog!

March 2020. An unprecedented time when the world stood still as Covid-19 wreaked havoc and transformed our way of life overnight.

What happened during the months that followed was hard to witness, difficult to understand and, I know, tragic for so many. There was uncertainty and confusion about what lay ahead, anxiety over this deadly virus and widespread loneliness as we were all forcibly separated from our familiar circles. There was collective grief for the loss in such a disempowering way. We were shown how vulnerable our structured mechanisms were and how powerless we were as individuals and society in dealing with the magnitude of such a global threat.

Dave found lockdown gruelling. Stifling. How do you confine a restless man in a small space? Answer: with enormous difficulty. All his work commitments came to a shuddering halt, filming and travel were not possible and life morphed into a shape we didn't recognise. The boys' nationwide three-month tour scheduled for the autumn was cancelled, which was heartbreaking for them – Dave struggled with having no project to focus on and nothing to plough his creativity into. He had always been free to roam and explore – this was a man who craved excitement and experience. Suddenly, he'd had his wings clipped and was at home with nothing to do but twiddle his thumbs and no sign of anything exciting on the horizon.

We did have many reasons to be grateful though. We were financially secure, we had a comfortable roof over our heads with outdoor space and we had each other, unlike some poor souls who were forced into isolation alone.

Something else, too. A couple of weeks before lockdown, Dave had been into hospital for a cardiological procedure – he needed an ablation to treat an atrial-fibrillation or an irregular heart rhythm, which he amusingly described as 'doing the plumbing and electrics on my heart'. It all went as smoothly as possible and with hindsight he was very lucky to have had that medical attention right when he needed it, considering Covid was lurking just around the corner and about to bring our overstretched NHS to its knees.

* * *

I had lost my dad five months before the virus took hold and Dave and I had booked for my mum, who was grieving her loss, to fly over for a three-week holiday with us in Kent where we'd moved to from Barrow in 2016 for easier access to France.

She had been due to fly back home to Romania on 20 March, the same day all flights out of the UK were cancelled, a move swiftly followed by the then prime minister Boris Johnson's announcement of a nationwide lockdown, which meant no one would be flying anywhere for the foreseeable.

So, she was stuck with us. It proved to be an interesting situation with some very colourful and, at times, hilarious episodes. I could see how desperate Dave was for something to get his teeth into, which is why I suggested he did some cooking and baking videos and post them online, an idea he leapt upon and ran with. He needed to be doing something constructive and which kept him in touch with his audience. This was it.

With me behind the camera, we started filming in what Dave called his 'isolation kitchen', demonstrating how to make delicious dishes such as beef pot roast and wild garlic pasta with garlic he'd foraged on his permitted daily hour of exercise.

He once even challenged the Romanian ambassador to the UK, Dan Mihalache, to a culinary duel, with Dave barbecuing Romanian sausages called *mici* and the ambassador cooking a polenta dish. The challenge was then passed to the British ambassador in Bucharest and continued in a chain to other officials.

Dave would often film alongside my mum and the two of them developed this highly entertaining dynamic, mimicking or hand-gesturing towards each other with wooden spoons or rolling pins. The public loved those videos because it became clear very quickly that my mum couldn't and indeed wouldn't follow Dave's instructions. Imagine the scene. She didn't speak any English. He didn't speak any Romanian.

Mum had her own way of doing things and Dave would have to stand aside, watching whatever she was trying to do with the food he'd just prepared. If he wanted his oxtail ravioli cut one way, you can bet your bottom dollar that my mum had other ideas and would bat his hand away if he tried to intervene. I remember one time she physically pushed him aside and took over the prep because she didn't agree with the way he was handling the rolling pin and the dough.

I'm overjoyed that we captured so much of this on camera.

There were many times when Dave, always the perfectionist, didn't like the results of their joint enterprise and would bin whatever they'd just cooked. My mum would be outraged about the waste.

'This dish is all right!' she'd exclaim.

'It has to be more than all right,' said Dave. 'It must be perfect. And if it's not perfect, it's not good enough for us.'

At times, I didn't dare translate what they were saying to each other! Having my mum with us through all those months actually helped us because at least we didn't have the worry of her going through lockdown alone at home in Romania. She was safe with us, we could take care of her while Dave, whose focus was on keeping her well, made sure she had all her usual medication sent to the UK.

It wasn't easy for her though and every day she'd make me check online to see if there were any flights, desperately homesick, missing her church and its tight-knit community. She was also feeling sorry for her garden back home, which needed all the spring prep work done in time for the summer, and I'd sometimes find her crying, deeply unhappy, not knowing what to do with herself.

To help ease some of her sadness, I went online and ordered shelves, trays, bags of soil, seeds and bulbs, and created a small veggie patch in the corner of our courtyard for her to potter about with. I also got her a tablet and installed a live connection to her local church sermons so she could virtually attend every Sunday and chat to some of her friends. All this helped to lift her mood enormously and she started to smile again. The internet was quite the magic pill for upset in those days, wasn't it?

We adapted our life to her preferences and because she liked to be in bed by seven, we got used to eating dinner much earlier than in normal times, and the meals Dave prepared were tailored to her tastes. The food where we come from is very limited and not remotely fancy, and so my mum is not what you'd call a culinary daredevil. She was used to survival food and survival food was the opposite of what Dave normally dished up. My mum was happy enough with the basics, but Dave only ever wanted the best. He was so thoughtful with what he cooked, mindful that my mum and her palate would not be ready for his more extravagant creations. But he did push her ever so gently into trying new flavours and textures, and as a result she became a little more experimental, a little more daring, starting to enjoy foods she'd never tried before.

I remember her having her first prawn, just as I had done many years before when I moved to Barrow. The only fish we get back home is either tinned or trout, and there was some-thing endearing about watching her taste buds come alive. Oh, and she was head over heels for the fish and chips the way Dave did them. He took such great care with his chips, which had to be – you got it – perfect. They'd be cut the same length, not thin but not too chunky either, and then triple-cooked until they were crisp and golden. He'd then build them like bricks, forming a grid on the plate, and only after that did he add the fish, placing the pieces – all the same size – gently alongside.

He used to say, 'We eat with our eyes first,' so took as much care with the presentation as he did the cooking. It had to be as visually appealing as it was delicious. Mum loved to sit and watch Dave cook – seeing a man in the kitchen was a revelation to her.

It was hardly surprising that food was the common denominator when it came to keeping up Dave's spirits. We couldn't see the kids in person and so in order to keep the family engaged and active, he'd plan dinners together, ordering us the same fine-dining boxes to be delivered from restaurants and then setting up a date when all of us would eat together on Zoom. Of course, all this food had to be accompanied with good wine. Having had to cope with my dad's drinking habits for the whole of their married life, my mum was very alcohol averse and would wave her finger reproachfully whenever she saw bottles and glasses on the table. Dave and I would wait for her to retire to bed before cracking open the vino – what she couldn't see couldn't hurt her, after all.

I suppose boozing was a soothing habit many people turned to during those lockdown evenings, a temporary numbing effect of the pain and anxious thoughts and a short-term mood enhancement to boot. Dave and I were no different and we'd order boxes of wine online, asking the couriers to leave them by the gate to hide them from my mum's disapproving eyes. We'd then have to dispose of the empty bottles without her noticing and it became a little game for Dave and me, making us giggle like naughty teenagers.

We also started working our way through a lot of TV series – *Peaky Blinders* was a favourite – but Dave would usually fall asleep after one or two episodes and then get cross with me if I continued watching without him. The next evening I'd have to flick through every scene until he determined where he'd lost the plot the night before and then rewatch it all again with him.

One evening, after the usual process of setting the table, eating a lovely dinner and then my mum going to bed, we opened a bottle and started watching *Hunters*, a conspiracy thriller set in seventies New York, which starred Al Pacino and was about a squad chasing down former Nazi officers to bring them to justice. After a couple of glasses of wine, Dave disappeared up to the bedroom. I knew he was up to something, I could feel it.

Sure enough, half an hour later and having been inspired by a character in the series, he reappeared in a 'ta-dah!' moment with a freshly groomed goatee-style beard, looking not unlike a seventies porn star. It looked *ridiculous* on him, but it was bloody hilarious and we laughed for days at his impromptu makeover which he decided to keep.

It was a drunken impulse he carried into the series *Hairy Bikers Go North*, which the boys filmed later in 2020 as soon as it was possible for them to go back to work.

* * *

Our house in Kent was very modern and full of electronic gadgets and gizmos. Annoyingly, we depended on the tech for everything and while it was *supposed* to make life easier, not even the simple task of drawing the curtains was a straightforward process. There was a data room in the basement housing the cables, devices, processors, motors, drivers and numerous other objects that were beyond our comprehension. There was always some sort of a fight with technology, challenging our skills and testing our patience.

One day, this room overheated from all the intense electrical activity and it affected the engine that activated the mechanism to draw the curtains. This being lockdown, we couldn't call anyone to assist and it took Dave quite a while (and a few burst fuses of his own) to figure out what the problem was. But he did it! His fingers were bleeding and his face was covered in sweat, but his pride was intact. And that night we could draw the curtains. Such was Dave's determination; when he put his mind into things, he usually succeeded. Eventually.

Then there was the garden. We had a small lawn at the back of the house that Dave used to describe as 'the Serengeti' due to its propensity for weeds, which would spike up between the blades of grass. He wanted it to look 'lush and perfectly smooth, just like velvet' and lockdown gave him the time to devote to this mission.

Dave spent many, *many* hours crawling on the grass using tweezers and scissors to reach the parts a mower could not and to pick out the dandelions and clover leaves one by one. Unfortunately, our Westie Dougie, who had arrived in our family as a playmate for Snowy in 2015, didn't appreciate the efforts … or maybe he appreciated them a bit too much. Dave would despair at the number of times a back leg was cocked to pee all over his tireless work. Such disrespect! I'd hear the expletives coming from the garden and know Dougie had been up to his tricks again.

I kept myself busy too. I had an urge to be useful and to do something to help and it all happened quite spontaneously after news emerged that hospitals were lacking personal protective equipment (PPE) for staff. There was a lot of discussion on various Facebook groups about organising something for the NHS and a bunch of us got our heads together to form a network of sewing enthusiasts from across the country, all eager to lend their skills and donate their time. For those NHS workers who were putting themselves in front of this illness, this felt like the least I could do in return.

We swung into action, sourcing the correct NHS-approved blue cotton fabric used for scrubs – there was a company in Preston who donated and delivered about 1,000 metres of fabric, which I then distributed within the group. We made hats, masks and sets of scrubs, and Dave took on the role of my glamorous assistant, modelling the finished garments so we could post pictures on social media and encourage more people to join our collective.

We were in touch with personnel on the ground at the hospitals, so we knew who needed what and we quickly became a powerful force, this little cottage industry serving the NHS. Once there was a batch of items ready to be delivered, the biking group Volunteer Riders UK would come and pick up the parcels and take them where they needed to go. Dave always enjoyed a socially distanced chat about bikes with the guys who dropped by to collect.

None of us in the group had met each other before and yet we managed to create something quite remarkable together. I met a few of them after lockdown was over and it was lovely to put faces to names. I still have friends from those times.

Dave and Me

Despite all the trauma Covid brought, I believe something else transpired as a result. As people, we proved more resourceful than we thought possible, and the way communities came together was inspirational and life-affirming. Where there was separation, there was also unity and connection. Where there was suffering, there would be someone or something to bring consolation.

It was also during lockdown that I finally achieved a long-held ambition to qualify as a coach and hypnotherapist. There were so many people I knew who were lost during that turbulent time and I wanted to do something productive.

I signed up for some online courses and started a virtual group which met every Sunday for an hour, a platform for people to share what was happening to them and a chance to do some meditation together. As well as Britain, we had members from Italy, France, Canada and America, and it was such a lovely way to meet people and release some anxiety about what was going on in the world. There were some beautiful moments. I carried on with my training after lockdown and, when it was allowed again, completed some in-person courses. It's a constant privilege to host a space for someone to talk and to help them see their situation from a different angle. Changing the perspective even just slightly can open up a whole heap of other possibilities.

Dave missed Si during the months stuck at home, although they started work on a new book and began doing a weekly live together on Instagram, which was popular with the Hairy

Bikers community and beyond. Sometimes they'd do a cook-along with simple recipes made from everyday ingredients, other times they'd just tell stories or answer questions people had sent in. With great affection, Dave would say, 'Now it's time for me to speak to my disciples', and he loved to see people's comments and the reactions on the screen, especially when the heart emojis flooded in. Those interactions would be the inspiration for the podcast, *Agony Uncles*, which the boys launched in 2022, a series of 30–40-minute episodes giving people often hilarious advice on questions related to different life challenges.

When Covid restrictions eased enough for filming projects to resume, Dave headed off in the autumn of 2020 to shoot *Hairy Bikers Go North* and it was like he'd escaped from prison. He was liberated! He and Si hit the road travelling across the North of England, sampling and showcasing the best northern grub they could find. Covid hadn't disappeared by any means and they had to be cautious about where they filmed and of other people. I was worried about him and he did contract Covid the following year which affected him very badly. He couldn't breathe properly and had to miss all the promotion engagements for the series which started on BBC Two in September 2021. Si had to go it alone. We had no idea that Covid would soon be the least of our concerns. And nothing compared to the health challenges and heart-ache that were to come.

The Shoes

30 November 2024

Today is a big day for me, something I've been building myself up for. Over these last months, not only have I had to mourn my man, but I've also had to come out of my shell.

When Dave was alive he protected us, his family, as much as possible from any intrusion or media attention. That wasn't our world. We'd occasionally step into it and enjoyed some of the perks, but the spotlight was always Dave's domain and he occupied it so well.

That's changed now and I have been making myself step up and talk publicly about Dave, whether in front of press and TV cameras or from behind a radio microphone, in the hope that others might be inspired to share their feelings of loss too. Stepping up has also meant finding the courage to attend high-profile events without him and so this evening I'm going to a Christmas ball at the London Marriott Hotel organised by the Romanian community, which this year is dedicated to the life and legacy of Dave. He loved everything about my country and before his illness we'd done a lot to support different Romanian charities or individuals, or events organised by the community in the UK.

For a number of years, we attended this Romanian Gala event every Christmas and how I wish he was coming with me tonight, getting ready to dance the night away as he had done in the past. Instead, I'm being accompanied by my family and some beautiful friends who have all been my rocks throughout the last year. My best friend, Anna, has come over and is bringing her orchestra of classical musicians from Paris to perform on the night.

Nevertheless, I want to find a way of taking Dave with me and so I'm looking through my wardrobe, trying to find something of significance to take to the ball. All these lovely dresses he bought for me or encouraged me to make for myself, each one with a story to tell about a place or an event he was invited to with me as his plus one. Tonight though, he is my plus one! So I'm searching for something – or some things – that will bring a bit of Dave to the party.

And here they are.

Two boxes. Two separate Christmas presents from Dave, both full of the same playful spirit. Before I reveal their contents, I must tell you about how Christmases are … were … celebrated in our family. In Eastern Europe, the traditional Christmas meal happens on Christmas Eve, so that's how Dave and I did it too. We'd have dinner (usually pork) and drinks before heading to the nearest church for the midnight service. On returning home at about 1am, everyone would exchange gifts and we'd eventually go to bed around four. Tired after such a long, late night, most of us stayed in bed on Christmas morning, although Dave would be dashing about the kitchen cooking the turkey and a traditional British Christmas dinner with all the trimmings and sauces, ready to go again for round two.

He would go above and beyond to make it special – I mean, we all enjoyed Christmas, but Dave? He LOVED it. The decorations, the banter, the cooking, the music, the *mess* and the kitchen sink overflowing with dirty dishes scraped clean, all of it was sheer pleasure for him.

One year, when my parents were over and we had other guests staying too, he very mischievously convinced my dad to wear an elf suit because 'in Britain all men dress up for Christmas'. That year, the turkey was served by Dave wearing a mankini. A sight not forgotten in a hurry!

The gift-giving was Dave's icing on the Christmas cake. He always took care to buy us the most unusual and creative presents.

Which brings me to the two boxes I'm looking at right now.

Both of them bear the Dolce & Gabbana logo. The smaller box is particularly special and it makes me laugh just looking at it. Dave handed it to me on Christmas Eve 2022, so proud of himself. I slowly lifted the lid, appreciating the moment, to find inside the most stunning, jewel-adorned D&G bag ... um, handle.

Dave's face dropped. He thought he'd bought me the whole handbag, but it was only a replacement handle for a specific model. Well, the whole lot of us burst out laughing when we realised what had happened. Poor Dave! He'd meant well and had a heart of gold so I could see the disappointment on his face. I assured him that this was a sign for me to create the perfect bag for this perfect handle and a few months later I did just that.

So now I have an elaborate handmade bag to go with my elaborate D&G bag handle and the whole piece is completely unique – problem solved!

Inside the second box is a pair of shoes that Dave gave me for Christmas 2019, just before the pandemic started. They're gorgeous and sparkly, covered in silver sequins and colourful buckles with red, green and golden stones. I'd never seen such a sensational pair of shoes before and I remember when I opened the box thinking that they deserved to be put in a glass display, never to be worn but forever admired.

As I look at them now, it brings back warm memories of times when things were good and we were happy. Dave rarely spent money on himself but loved spending it on me and he'd always push me to treat myself with expensive goodies.

He could be very romantic and if he was ever working away over Valentine's, he'd make sure there was a massive bunch of flowers and balloons delivered to the house. One year they were delivered to my neighbour across the road by mistake and she came over with them later.

'I thought they were for me!' she said. 'I thought *finally* my husband's sent me flowers for Valentine's, but no. You're a lucky girl, Lil!'

But it wasn't just gifts he showered me with, it was love, attention and humour. He could be very cheeky as well, mind. And jolly inappropriate. The Bikers were once filming on a farm and he had to milk a goat.

'This one's just like my wife,' he said, 'one tit bigger than the other!'

Ha! Perhaps not quite the way you'd want your husband to describe you on TV, but it made me laugh – Dave was a sunny-side-up kind of guy who possessed a young-at-heart desire to find the fun in everything … even if he was likening me to a goat.

My eyes fall upon an envelope in the shoe box, something I'd forgotten about completely, and when I pick it up and turn it around, my heart sinks.

His handwriting.

His quirky way of saying things to make me love him more.

'To my dearest Liliana, I love you. I really am your sugar daddy!'

Oh, Dave.

I've only worn these shoes once before and that was at his funeral. I'd wanted everyone to wear something 'Dave' that day, an item of clothing that was just as colourful and eccentric as he had been his whole life. The shoes were my personal tribute to him, a way to show myself and the world that I was honouring his life with a smile on my face. A brave face. And with a pain in my heart that no one could ever understand.

It's decided. These most epic of shoes and the homemade handbag with its dazzling handle are coming to the Christmas ball with me. They are so very Dave and such a reflection of the way I feel right now that it seems entirely fitting to wear them with pride. As I leave the house to catch my train to London, I know they will serve to make me stronger and more visible tonight.

Together they will tell a story – my story – of deep love and immense grief that I choose to carry with me with grace and integrity.

Chapter Ten

Diagnosis

Look at Si, he's chopping away like Keith Richards at a party!

When the phone call came through on the car's dash display, I recognised the London code and knew instantly it was Dave's doctor.

I also sensed that this wasn't going to be good news.

I was right.

'David,' said the doctor, getting straight to the point, 'I'm sorry to tell you that you have cancer. You'd better come to my office as soon as possible so we can start planning for treatment.'

From that moment, nothing would ever be the same again.

It was the end of March 2022 and Dave and I were driving through Normandy to our home in France for a two-week trip. We'd been so looking forward to this time away where we planned to tackle the garden, but our hearts were heavy as we'd just heard that Dave's cousin Les had died.

Car journeys to and from France were normally accompanied by a Milly Johnson audiobook, but given the news about Les, neither of us were able to focus enough to listen. Instead, we'd been talking about Les, his wife Muriel, their life together working on the shipyard in Barrow and how much Dave admired them.

We always shared the driving and it was my turn behind the wheel. I remember being extra cautious on the road because the conditions outside were dark and wet.

Then came the call that changed everything.

We'd both had our annual general check-ups in January, the usual tests to make sure everything was as it should be. Dave hadn't been feeling quite right in the run-up to his and had asked the doctor to run a few tests besides the routine. Initial results indicated there was nothing to worry about, which had reassured us enough to head to France, but it was the last batch that the doctor was now phoning about.

Dave listened to what he was told about the next steps, too shocked to form a coherent response. By now we were only about an hour from the French house, so we didn't stop or turn back, just continued the journey in a stunned silence. Neither of us knew what to say. We spent the next four days hiding away, putting off returning to the UK, allowing the news to sink in. We cried a lot, took long walks in places we'd never been before and where we were guaranteed not to meet anyone.

Deserted places, just like our souls in those moments.

Reeling and in a state of disbelief, we mourned our unfinished plans, our unfulfilled hopes, and discussed at length how this was going to affect us, our family, friendships, work, our whole world. How it was going to take over our lives in ways we could not yet conceive and how out of control of his own life Dave suddenly felt.

We didn't eat, barely slept, both disorientated and drifting like ships without a compass. After a couple of days, we called Si and Dr Dave to tell them the news and those were very hard, distressing conversations to have. We didn't tell the kids until we got back to the UK when we organised a Zoom call with them. I don't have any memories about driving back, the journey to a reality neither of us wanted to face.

Dave was referred to a specialist and on the Monday morning – just six days after we'd received that phone call from the doctor – he went to have the port installed into an artery in his chest ready to start chemotherapy the following day. It was all so quick and he struggled – as did I – to come to terms with what was happening.

'I've just got to a point in my life when I've achieved everything I ever wanted,' he'd say, 'and now I feel it's all being taken away in such a brutal way. I've got a loving family, a place I can call home and a dream of a career. Why? Oh why? Where have I gone wrong?'

I couldn't answer those questions. Acceptance felt like an impossibility and the feeling of a sharp knife in the pit of my stomach was something I could not shake off. My hair turned completely white within a couple of weeks of Dave's diagnosis and my nights were restless.

Over the next three months, his treatment was very aggressive and the side effects were debilitating and ugly. It got to the point where he was too ill to speak; after each bout, one of the substances he was being given brought on a temporary speech impediment so he could not properly articulate words. He had sores in his mouth which meant he was unable to eat or drink and was suffering with such severe nerve damage in his hands that he had to wear gloves. He had it in his legs too, which affected his balance and ability to walk. I remember Si picked us up from the hospital one day and he was shocked at the state of Dave, who was a shadow of his former self.

Losing his hair as a result of the chemo was incredibly painful for Dave given his history of alopecia and the regrowth following the surgery in 1998 for the arachnoid cyst. The decision to shave it all off was our way of taking control, which was psychologically beneficial, although it took him a while to get used to being bald again. He felt reduced to being only a cancer patient, stripped of his image, identity and personality, and with a face he no longer recognised.

He told me how difficult he found it to love himself when he looked in the mirror because the physical change was so drastic. He thought he was hideous with no hair, no eyelashes and heavily stained teeth from chemo. He'd lost a lot of muscle mass which meant his skin sagged, the neuro-pathy in his hands and feet made them unbearably achy, and some fingernails and toenails had fallen off.

Dave and Me

He found himself repellent.

The hair loss also made Dave's illness very visible and although his wish would have been to deal with things privately, he knew as a public figure that it wouldn't be long before the news got out. He decided to tell people in a typically honest, human way, without fuss or fanfare, and it made sense to drop it into conversation on the *Agony Uncles* podcast, keeping details about his treatment vague and saying nothing of the prognosis or the type of cancer, a decision I am honouring in this book.

He told listeners he would be stepping back from filming commitments for a while but was 'cracking on' and remaining upbeat. The podcast had become important to Dave and he would build himself up and draw on what little strength he had for the boys' one-hour recording. For the rest of the week he would be very poorly indeed.

It was always the two days following chemo that were the worst. After that, he would have a marginal recovery, getting better towards the end of the week, only to have to start all over again. We had to learn how to navigate this vicious cycle as best we could. In those months of turmoil, we talked about the past, the places we loved visiting, our achievements, our regrets, the lessons we'd learned in our lives and the ones we would like to pass on to our children. We spoke about the things he would have loved to have done but had not yet got round to. And the things he had done before but now wouldn't be able to.

Losing his appetite for cooking and eating made him deeply depressed. Food had always been such a central piece of Dave's existence; without it he didn't know who he was anymore.

Going back to the food we ate in childhood is normal in difficult moments and this is what Dave did, adopting familiar and comforting ways of eating such as shepherd's pie or tins of Heinz soup. But this was also upsetting for him, having acquired so much experience and knowledge and then returning to his roots. It was as if everything he'd built up through passion and hard work had melted away, turned into dust by an invasive treatment that was supposed to help control the cancer.

He told me about his fears. Fears that people wouldn't listen to him anymore, because he was 'damaged'.

That the cancer would mean he was discarded and forgotten.

That he would die in pain.

In those moments, my heart would plummet and I'd hold him, wrapping my arms around him tightly so he could feel my heartbeat and my love.

My heartbreak and my pain.

There wasn't much I could say to provide any comfort except that I was there for him and wasn't going anywhere.

We both knew what was coming. Dave had been in my shoes years before when he'd lost Glen and I had to have a realistic view of what lay ahead. I'm a practical person by nature and there was a moment when I had to make a decision about what the immediate future was going to look like. I had a choice between crying and despairing at Dave's suffering or stepping up to do what was necessary to keep us both afloat. I chose to step up, with all the determination I could muster. I'm sure people who have been through similar journeys know exactly what I'm talking about. Carers do what must be done.

I took steps towards creating a new normality and bringing back a bit of hope, making adaptations in the house and addressing the food patterns. Chemo had completely altered his taste buds but he barely had any appetite anyway and we were fighting an uphill battle to make sure he took in enough calories to keep his weakened body going. I started to prepare fresh juices, smoothies, soups – foods he could easily swallow. But even those were not easy for him to consume.

Sleep was difficult as well, because he couldn't stand anything touching his feet, not even a light bedsheet. Even the merest pressure created stabs of pain and I had to change our bedding and his pyjamas to the softest cotton I could find. T-shirts were worn inside out so the seams would not rub against and irritate his skin. Socks, once such a thing of joy for Dave, his jazzy collection so intrinsic to his sense of style, would leave painful grooves on his shins so I searched in many shops trying to find loose knitted pairs that wouldn't hurt as much.

His physical pain and low self-esteem made him avoid socialising, but I'd occasionally organise visits from friends so he could see he wasn't alone. I focused every effort on making the treatment as bearable as possible. There were times when family and friends stepped in to help with the various logistics, which eased the burden for me. Sergiu, Iza and her partner, Emilio, took turns to come and collect us from the hospital in London. Si, Dr Dave and our friend Armen Lloyd were all there in a heartbeat whenever we needed them. They were rocks for us.

Between treatments during the day Dave would watch TV, which proved an effective distraction, and he developed a routine that started with *BBC Breakfast*, then moved on to *Homes Under the Hammer*, *Antiques Roadshow*, *Classic Cars* and *The Chase*. Sometimes he would turn to the cookery channels to watch reruns of old Hairy Bikers' series and I'd see tears form in his eyes. When he noticed, he'd quickly switch over.

My training in coaching and hypnotherapy gave me a toolbox of coping mechanisms and having my community of helpers and healers at hand was life-saving for me. There were people available whenever I needed to offload and I was supported in many ways to find my own strategies. The same help was available to Dave, but his faith in that kind of support was not strong. He was much more comfortable talking to a psychologist when we finally got access to one, and their phone and Zoom conversations did seem to bring him some relief.

Nevertheless, I recorded him a short and relaxing piece of meditation that he could listen to before sleep, with soft music and my voice whispering calmly and peacefully, placing him at Lake Geneva, one of his favourite places we'd visited together.

I promised to take him back there when he was feeling better – this was a promise I would be able, thankfully, to keep.

* * *

It so happened that at the time of Dave starting treatment we were in the process of moving house from Kent to Staffordshire, near Burton-on-Trent. Long before his diagnosis, Dave had felt a pull to move further north and after a few unfruitful viewings around the Cheshire area, he'd spotted a house he liked online in the autumn of 2021.

It was in a lovely tranquil spot in Staffordshire and halfway between Manchester and the Cotswolds where Iza and Sergiu respectively lived. Our offer was accepted and, after putting the Kent house on the market, we became part of a large, precarious chain for the next nine months. By the time we eventually moved in July 2022, Dave was three months into his treatment. It was also when his medical team in London delivered the devastating news that the treatment was not working in our favour.

I had wanted to pull out of the house move, thinking it was too much to bear given everything else we were dealing with, but Dave was adamant that we go ahead. To him the Kent house, which had suffered a couple of floods, meant trouble and illness and he wanted to turn the page. We had also found the weekly Kent to London commute for Dave's chemo a real struggle. There were no parking spaces at the hospital so that meant taking a train the night before, staying in a hotel, getting a taxi to the hospital at 8am for the blood draw, waiting for the results to show the count was all right, remaining there for the treatment and then relying on family or friends to come and take us home. The alternative was to travel back by train during rush hour, something we did end up having to do a couple of times, and it was horrible to see Dave so ill walking the platforms, his veins filled with radio-active substances.

One day we'd hired a taxi to take us straight home, but the car suffered a puncture on the way and a two-hour journey took us five. The travelling was exhausting and painful for both of us and we needed a change. That change came with the move to Staffordshire because it also meant switching hospitals.

Si came to help look after Dave as I packed up the Kent house and headed to the new one. The boys stayed in a B&B while I made sure there was a comfortable bedroom set up for Dave who arrived in Staffordshire the next day, driven by Si in Dave's car. And that was our move back up north complete.

'I don't remember buying a house with stairs,' was Dave's first comment when he arrived at the new house. He needed support to climb the ten steps to the front door. Our new home was actually a large apartment in a big Victorian building with a history connected to the beer industry. I guess that was one of the major selling points for Dave when he'd viewed it the year before.

It was a fabulous place with high ceilings, sash windows and spacious rooms, organised around a former internal courtyard, which now has a glass roof and floods the space with light. I styled this central part of the house with sitting areas and indoor plants and it became our 'orangery'.

In moments of anguish, Dave and I would lay down on the floor there, watching the blue sky through the glass. We'd see birds flying overhead or the occasional small plane heading towards the airfield nearby, glimpses of life in the sky above us.

The rest of the world continued while ours had stopped turning.

We'd hold hands and cry, sometimes unable to move or talk, just despairing at the unfairness of it all. We both fought through many dark moments together and many more separately. I could feel his pain, I knew so well the depth of it, the desperation, the helplessness, the anger. Desperation for the loss of the peace and safety we'd both worked so hard for and would never get back. Helplessness in the face of this invisible enemy we'd been told was going to conquer us, no matter what we did or tried. Anger at the injustice of having his life cut short and for being dragged through all this pain, the hospital appointments and the invasive treatments, knowing there was no way out.

There were still so many things he wanted to do, so much work planned in his head and so many more adventures we'd dreamed of having together.

People used to tell him how brave he was, but what choice did he have? What choice did we have other than to keep going, listen to the specialists and hope for the best? But throughout all these dreadful months, the love was there. Loving someone doesn't stop when you, or they, are at their lowest point. Love doesn't switch off when they are weak and broken and rely on you for everything. We were together through thick and thin, in sickness and health, we trusted each other in every aspect of our relationship and in the most loving, truthful, beautiful way.

Dave would say, 'This isn't fair on you, Lil ...' and I'd tell him I would not be anywhere else in the world. Being there and taking care of him was what my love for Dave and my commitment to our marriage meant. Watching over him during that extraordinarily painful time in our lives was what I wanted to do.

Was it easy? Of course not.

Was it without its frustrations? Hell, no.

Dave could be an awkward patient at times and I often felt ill-equipped to care for him or to know what to do. He was a proud man and made every effort to look after his personal hygiene, rejecting my help there, but he relied on me for just about everything else. His weakened muscles and problematic balance made walking quite difficult, but he refused to use the walking sticks I bought him in the house, let alone in public.

That meant he had to lean on my arm all the time to avoid falling and it took us a while to suss out a safe way to do this for us both. How to walk, how to get up or down stairs, how to lift him off a bed or a chair, how to get in and out of the car. Simple everyday actions that you don't realise the importance of until they become impossible.

But despite my misgivings about the move, Dave had been right about the need for a change and it wasn't long before we were both feeling the benefit. It made a huge difference to us that The Priory Hospital in Birmingham was about 30 miles away from where we'd moved to. I'd drive him in, park the car, stay with him during treatment and then drive him home in the evening. The travelling was a doddle compared to London and this would be our lives for the next 18 months with at least one trip a week to the hospital and/or the physio.

Dave's physiotherapy at Circle Rehabilitation Birmingham was a saviour for him. His balance improved as did his confidence and, remarkably, within the space of a few weeks, he could walk on his own without having to lean on my arm.

He would arrive for his 'go-go juice', as he called the treatment, in good spirits. He knew all of the nurses by name and enjoyed the banter and endless chat about food, recipes, ingredients. There was always a friendly face checking up on us and a good cup of tea – some nurses even baked at home and brought the goods into the hospital for Dave to taste.

There was Guia who cooked him a tasty Filipino noodle dish called *pancit*, one of the few things Dave fancied eating

– he even included it in the last Christmas special the boys filmed towards the end of 2023. Marion, a lovely Irish nurse, baked him a cheesecake for his 66th birthday in September 2023 when all the staff on the ward came in to surprise him, singing 'Happy Birthday' while he was tethered to the drips.

We didn't know it then, but that was to be Dave's last birthday and I can't thank those beautiful ladies enough for their kindness in such vulnerable times for us.

We had also started putting building blocks in place to boost Dave's confidence, which had taken a real pummelling – this man who had once been so gregarious and uninhibited was now diminished and withdrawn. I wanted him to find the courage to live again, to see that he could have moments of normality or excitement and that we were still able to create memories as a family, or for him to enjoy on his own.

When the boys were invited to the Queen's Platinum Jubilee celebrations to be part of the pageant on an open-top bus through the streets of London in the summer of 2022, Dave's initial response had been to turn it down.

'No, I'm not going. Look at me, I look like an egg! I can't go like this.'

'Darling,' I replied, 'you are going. Even if I have to carry you, I'm taking you there.'

I wholeheartedly admit to being pushy because I knew that if he was going to have any quality of life then he needed to be forced out of what had become his comfort zone: the house, the sofa and the remote control.

So, wearing a jaunty orange hat, a smart blazer and tie, he went to the Jubilee and he got on that bus. Along with Si and a host of other celebrities and sports stars, he ended up thoroughly enjoying himself, just as I'd known he would. The more he got out there, the more confidence he gained, so I continued to encourage him

For Dave's 65th birthday, shortly after starting treatment in Birmingham, Sergiu booked dinner for us all at Lunar, a terrific restaurant in Stoke-on-Trent. Dave was very nervous about that night and being seen out in public, unsteady on his feet and with no hair, but it all went smoothly and even though he couldn't eat much, he really appreciated being sat at a nice table in a special place with the people who loved him most.

Beforehand he had been afraid of being recognised 'looking like a freak' – he was used to being approached in restaurants; people would ask for selfies or for his opinion on the food. At the very least he'd get a good-natured yell of, 'Where's your bike?'

But it didn't happen this time, which in turn caused him to have a brief moment of, 'Oh, so I'm a nobody now ...' I think Dave felt conflicted. There was relief at not being spotted but also the stark realisation that he was now so unrecognisable no one noticed him. Personally, I was glad that he could spend time with us anonymously without having to feel obliged to talk to curious strangers whilst being so vulnerable.

Buoyed by that successful dinner out, I booked him on an hour-long flight with the local flying club. I anticipated some resistance from Dave so didn't tell him my plan until the day itself, breaking the news to him in the car on the way there. Predictably, he reacted badly.

'I'm not able to walk properly and you want me to fly? There's no way chemo goes with flying an aeroplane. I can't do it.'

But he did it! He took so many photos as the pilot flew him over our house, above the area that we now called home. In the past Dave had a pilot's licence and before we met had done a lot of flying in his microlight. I knew he missed it because he'd told me so many times, which meant this experience was a real treat for him even if he didn't appreciate the surprise element. Dave Myers always liked to have a plan and it had to be one he'd created. Well, now it was my turn to make plans, to help him reclaim his *joie-de-vivre*.

My next one came from an idea we'd had in lockdown while watching the Dutch musician and conductor André Rieu's concerts on Sky Arts. Dave, who was healthy at that time, expressed a wish to go to Maastricht to attend one of Rieu's Christmas concerts and I made that possible in December 2022 when I bought tickets for us both. As Dave wouldn't countenance the idea of airports, I booked us on the Hull to Rotterdam overnight ferry, then drove from there to Maastricht for the annual show on Vrijthof Square.

The tickets included accommodation, transfers from hotel to the concert hall and back, plus a pre-concert dinner which was accompanied by some of the stars of Rieu's orchestra who played while we were dining. To our amazement, the top violinist, Cord Meyer-Luesink, recognised Dave and strode off the stage to come and ask for a picture with him.

How extraordinary was that?

He told us how he and his mother were big fans of the Hairy Bikers and I was deeply moved, grateful for this touching moment. The whole night was so uplifting for Dave and me as we were swept up in the festive spirit. And that was not all I'd planned.

From Maastricht, we travelled on to Brussels for a night near the Grand-Place. I mentioned earlier that years before, when Dave and I were still courting, we'd met there after the boys had finished filming and we'd both written secret wishes to hang on the Christmas tree. Today was the day my wish came true because we had returned to that square together … and how things had changed between then and now. Dave couldn't stand on his feet for too long, but we both felt it was right to be there again, watching the illuminations artfully projected onto the beautiful buildings. At one corner of the market we found a pub where I had a glass of champagne and Dave tried some local sausages.

The whole trip made him a bit more sure of himself – even optimistic – although he still wanted reassurance from the oncologist who was treating him at the Priory before he did anything at all. He liked her, trusted her opinion, and if she'd said he couldn't manage a journey like this, he would not have gone. Of that I am certain.

Pushing Dave to stretch himself was good for me, too. Taking him to good restaurants, to have him fly, to travel to our favourite places and to give him these moments, these glimmers while knowing that our time was limited, felt healing. Creating memories together was the right thing to do.

With that in mind, on 24 December 2022, I organised a big Christmas Eve dinner and invited all our new neighbours round for a feast of Romanian food. We'd always had fun hosting parties and Dave was over the moon to have people filling our home once more – the Staffordshire house was the perfect space for the lively gatherings we loved so much and we drank from crystal glasses while the open fire roared.

Our Christmases were always special, because Dave never held back with expense or extravagance and he went to town this year more than ever. We didn't have one Christmas tree, we had eight! All of them scattered around the ground-floor level. Our orangery resembled Santa's grotto and the dining room table was covered in baubles of all colours and shapes. What fun we had! That Christmas there was laughter and joy in our home again.

For us, the holiday season had always kicked off with a carol concert – we'd attended many organised by various charities we worked with over the years and when Iza was in the school choir we'd go and watch her perform at St Mary's Church in Dalton-in-Furness. And so another sign that Dave was feeling stronger was that he wanted to attend the Christmas sermon at the village church. Our local service was lovely and again, I felt gratitude for experiencing that with him as part of this community.

We were finishing 2022 in a stronger, more positive frame of mind than we had been just a few months before. The side effects of the new treatment were far milder and, combined with the physio and some good vitamins and supplements which helped his body recover and replenish, Dave was much more like his old self. He started making friends locally and the first one was Shummy, our local butcher. He loved going to Shummy's farm shop for banter while buying his favourite pieces of meat for our meals or exchanging opinions on recipes and methods of cooking. Dave was so happy living in the countryside and was grateful for the company of our neighbours who would often pop in for a bite to eat or a drink.

For the first time since his diagnosis, he managed to set foot in a TV studio at the invitation of Francois Gandolfi, the director the boys had worked with for years and who was now directing *Great British Menu*. Just being back on a set and feeling the flurries of activity and creative energy made Dave's eyes sparkle again, despite the fact that he had to rely on my arm for support to walk there. I loved seeing him so happy but at the same time I needed deep breaths to steady my thoughts. I wasn't going to kid myself.

We had mountains to climb and the bigger picture loomed terrifyingly large.

The Menu

2 December 2024

I'm in the garage, sorting through boxes we didn't get round to unpacking when we moved here two years ago. Back then my attention and focus were on caring for Dave, not on making this house our home. Nothing, not the wallpaper, carpets or lighting was chosen by us and part of me feels I let him down by neglecting all this.

In one of the boxes are two beautiful sconces that used to be in the lounge of the house in France and seeing them reminds me of how wonderful that room was. There's also a chandelier here, purchased in Bratislava on the same trip we bought our wedding rings, as well as various kitchen paraphernalia that I don't have a place for.

Now, *this* is interesting! In another box stuffed full of bits and bobs, I find a huge menu for L'Ancienne Auberge, a restaurant in the village of Vonnas, about 40 miles north of Lyon, where the fabulous chef Georges Blanc has held three Michelin stars since the mid-eighties. Dave liked to keep mementoes from various places he'd visited, but this menu is particularly sentimental. In 2016 the boys filmed a six-episode series called *Hairy Bikers Chicken and Egg,* which took them to countries such as Morocco, America and Israel in search of – correct! – the best chicken and egg recipes in the world.

Dave and Si's travels included a trip to eastern France and a region famous for its *poulet de Bresse,* a type of chicken known as the *crème de la crème* of French poultry. While there, they paid a visit to Georges' famous restaurant and learned how he prepared the bird, using methods passed down from his mother and grandmother. Dave was obsessed. The boys were literally salivating as Georges cooked this dish for them and, on the show, Dave said he was having a 'chicken-gasm' as he ate it! He returned from the trip describing the meal as 'the culinary experience of a lifetime'.

He couldn't wait to take me back there so he could show me what all the fuss was about, so shortly after filming wrapped, we went for a long weekend to Vonnas, booking a table at L'Ancienne Auberge. It was superb – everything Dave had promised it would be and more besides. To top it off, Georges, who was like royalty to Dave, came over to our table and signed this menu for us – 'For Dave and his love, thank you for coming to my restaurant' – and illustrated it with the picture of a cockerel.

Holding this menu now, I remember how chuffed Dave was with it and it makes my heart so happy. I can almost taste the meal we had that evening, such a simple dish of chicken breast with morels in a creamy sauce but done to absolute perfection.

Dave devoured it – he was always an 'enthusiastic' eater (to put it politely) and would often end up with a fair amount of the menu on his clothes – the sign, he would argue, of a good meal. He was audacious with food and would happily try anything put in front of him … apart from oysters which he always said 'make me a little bit untidy'.

He even tried goat's penis in Vietnam way back when the Hairy Bikers were filming their first series. Dave had spotted it on the menu and initially asked for two portions – one each for him and Si – but the waiter had laughed and advised, 'One is enough for two …' When the dish was brought to them, Si took 'the pointy end' and Dave took a ball.

'That was the first and the last time I'll have a penis in my mouth,' he told me later.

It seems unfathomably cruel and unfair that someone who embraced life with such an open heart and mind can be snatched away. Dave should have had decades left to fulfil his dreams and travel the world, to learn and soak up every second.

When I think like this, the survivor's guilt that lurks in my stomach can find its way to the surface. I know I'm by no means alone in feeling like this – it's an intense part of the maelstrom of hurt, pain and heaviness swirling inside us in the aftermath of losing someone we love. We feel that we should have been the ones taken instead, that we hadn't done enough before they passed and now we feel guilty for having time, when they have none, for living, when they are denied that.

That's exactly how I have felt – why do I deserve to live if life is without Dave? How can I justify 'life' on my own when he was denied his share? And when all my efforts to help him only proved my limited powers to find a way to keep him alive? In those dark moments, it was hard to think of all the joy I brought to his life. The love, the care, the devotion, they all fade unimportant in front of my inability to save him, to make things better for him.

'I, Lili Myers, was not able to take away my husband's pain and keep him alive. This is all my fault and therefore I have no worth.'

How good we are at blaming and shaming and beating ourselves up for things that are not, and never were, in our power. Why is it so difficult to accept the fact that we are not saviours and to acknowledge that we did the best we could? There's no way around the guilt unless you face it, so they say. With that in mind, I did quite a brave thing and painted mine, etching leaves and blades of grass onto a large canvas.

There is something about leaves when they break free from the branches in autumn and gently fall on the ground. The tree is stripped but grounded by its roots to withstand darker times until spring arrives with hope of a fresh start.

I've got to let my leaves fall, one by one, to get to the core of who I am without Dave. I must ground myself and find the promise of my new beginning. That was my painting.

My hand had moved across the canvas without me thinking, as if it was being led by an external force. I didn't interfere, I just let it happen, using a couple of leaves and blades of grass picked up on my walks with Teddy as inspiration. With every brushstroke came relief, which in turn started to break up the guilt as well.

I accept there were limits to what I was able to do. I know that my guilt is not helping me or the people around me. I learned to manage a situation that was out of my control and I can be proud of myself because I know I did everything humanly possible to make his life easier. It has taken me some time to acknowledge and understand those feelings and I am trying to practise self-compassion, talking openly to my support network about how I'm feeling.

I fish the Georges Blanc menu properly out of the box and dust it down.

It really is quite unique … far too special to be hidden away. It deserves to be seen! I make plans to frame it and hang it in an area of the house I'm creating for Dave.

This house that we chose together in better times, now so distant that they seem like lost dreams.

Chapter Eleven

Illness

Fry it until it's the colour of tramps' teeth!

The turn of the year – 2022 into 2023 – came with renewed energy and we dared to feel hopeful about life again. We were definitely in a better place.

Dave was a little bit more capable physically and his mood was much brighter. His appetite had returned, he'd started baking and cooking again, and had even bought himself a new bike. To take some of the pressure off before we moved house, he'd reluctantly sold a lot of them – we both had tears in our eyes when a van came to pick up the Moto Guzzi California we'd once travelled down to Italy on, back in the early days of courting. And the Laverda Jota, a collectors' item which Dave had lovingly restored over a number of years.

But in February 2023, he asked me to take him to Arnolds, the nearest bike shop to us in Burton-on-Trent, after something on their website had caught his eye. A bike he reckoned would be easy enough for him to handle.

What a triumph it was when I saw him wobbling towards it and then successfully mounting it in the shop. The look on his face! The beautiful olive-coloured Royal Enfield Bullet 500 Trials was delivered to him at home a few days later, and Dave named his new baby Gladys because encrusted in black on the number plate were the words, 'John loves Gladys'. We couldn't find any details as to who John and Gladys were, but the name stuck and Gladys is still in my garage to this day, ready for me to pass my motorbike licence and take her out on the road to freedom.

Being able to get on a bike once more and feel the engine revving gave Dave such a boost, adding to his overall well-being and our more upbeat outlook. He was managing to find gratitude for the little things and was appreciative of the time we spent together. His treatment at Birmingham was more bearable and as the daffodils began to sprout on our driveway and the birds started chirping again, it felt like a new dawn where anything might be possible.

He started doing a bit of online shopping for our new house, spending time on auction sites scouring for antiques, and he decorated our front living room with items full of character and history. A collection of Delft vases, a Royal Doulton potpourri dish, a Victorian coromandel sewing box – he'd research them all thoroughly before making his bid and it gave him so much pleasure to secure a piece he'd fallen in love with.

He was like a child opening his Christmas presents when they were delivered and our front room became an antique heaven, somewhere Dave loved to spend his evenings watching his favourite TV programmes while the fireplace danced with flames.

He bought two grandfather clocks, who he named Dudley and Jan, and he would set them off to chime against each other to 'give the house a heartbeat'. Dudley was a local 'lad', built in the late 1800s, while Jan was a Dutch senior from the eighteenth century. Whenever we had visitors, he would tell them the stories behind the objects with all of the old Dave gusto and I felt I had my husband back.

Spring had sprung and we enjoyed short walks in the nearby park. Dave's feet were not strong enough for long distances or uneven surfaces, so we'd regularly drive down to the lake where we'd sit and watch the geese on the water. Those days were very peaceful. In the middle of our village is a gated communal space with allotment plots and I took over one which helped us get out of the house a bit more often, to raise a bed or water seedlings. Back in healthier times, Dave had loved getting his hands dirty in our garden in France. Now even simple tasks were a lot more physically demanding, but when he needed a rest, he made a good assistant, sitting on a bench in the spring sun watching and giving me directions.

Life had steadied to a comfortable pace which allowed us to savour small pleasures – a world away from when Dave had started chemo and our days were so dark and brutal.

Around this time, there were talks about a potential project for a new Hairy Bikers series, the first since *Go North* which had been filmed between lockdowns and before Dave's diagnosis. This series was to be called *The Hairy Bikers Go West* and would see the boys exploring towns and suppliers along the UK's western coast. Dave and I talked at length about whether to take this on because his condition and treatment would require meticulous working around, both physically and logistically. He had appointments to attend and there would be days when his energy levels would be too low to work.

But mostly, Dave wanted to make sure I was OK with him spending periods of time away from home. Away from me. He was aware that we weren't certain about what the future held and that this was precious time for us. It would also mean that I'd only have him home for treatment days and then the recovery period immediately afterwards, not for any of the spells where he was on stronger form.

'Lil, what do you think about me going to film these months?' he asked. 'I won't accept this job if you don't want me to. I'd understand and respect your opinion.'

I believed him, but how could I say no when I knew how much it meant to him? When he had the chance, once again, to do what he loved and to feel normal and worthy again? To escape the agonising routine of hospitals, treatments and the harsh reality of this cruel illness? He wanted to be the person who made extraordinary things happen again. To connect with his public and also to convey a message that you can still have a life through cancer. It didn't have to stop everything.

Dave and Me

Although aware that this was shortening our time together, I encouraged him to go for it as long as provisions were made by the production company to care for his needs.

None of it was easy. On Thursdays Dave had chemo and would be in hospital all day. Fridays were mostly spent in bed with nausea and weakness. Saturdays tended to be a bit better and so he'd travel to the shoot location, then film across Sunday, Monday and Tuesday. On Wednesdays he'd travel home ready to start all over again the following day. I honestly don't know how he did it. How he found the mental and physical strength to get on this treadmill and deliver a whole series is beyond me.

In the past, Dave would never let me help him in his preparations for work or going away – I would do the laundry, ironing and folding, but that was it. His luggage was only for him to pack and always done as a strict routine. Having lived on the move throughout his career, what he had in his bag was crucial and therefore everything had a certain place, was packed in a particular order and I wasn't allowed to disrupt it.

Until now. Now he needed and accepted my help when it came to packing his bags.

'What do you think about this shirt, Lil? The blue one or the purple one? Which jacket should I take with me? I think the weather will be quite nice so maybe this lighter one?'

Those kinds of questions had always been rhetorical because he already knew exactly what he wanted. This time, however, he did listen to what I had to say.

The first day of filming was on the Isle of Bute, off the west coast of Scotland. I drove him to Seamill House Hotel in West Kilbride to join the crew – he was so nervous, yet so happy, and he'd managed the 300-mile journey north fairly comfortably, which reassured me this was going to be doable.

As we pulled into the hotel grounds, he spotted something that made him shriek with pleasure: his motorbike for the series. Eyes gleaming, he climbed out of the car and made his way towards it, circling it a few times to take in its beauty.

A BSA Gold Star.

It had undergone some alterations on the gear shifting pedal to accommodate Dave's restricted movement on his left leg caused by the neuropathy and I watched his face as he inspected every bit of it. I'd seen him do this many times in the past – when the two of them met their bikes for any forthcoming series it was with excitement, expectation and admiration. This was different, though. Just a few months before, Dave had thought he'd never have this chance again, so this was a moment to treasure.

He knew this would be his last series. We both knew.

There was a lot of help on set, made easier by the fact that it was the same crew who had been with the Hairy Bikers from more or less day one. Director Francois Gandolfi and cameraman Jon Boast were like Dave's second family, having been part of our lives and homes over many years.

South Shore, the production company, took great care to provide everything needed for Dave, even employing a nurse to be on the shoot. Si, too, was very protective over him and was the first one to make sure Dave had enough rest or food and that he was managing to keep pace with the shoot. The whole process must have been terribly hard emotionally for Si, seeing his friend going through this illness but finding the courage and strength to do it one last time, just like the old days.

Except it wasn't like the old days at all. Not for any of them. Their filming time was shorter than usual, their working days in the week were reduced and everything had to be built around Dave's physical capabilities. There was extra pressure, yet nobody complained; everybody did their very best to make things as easy as possible for Dave.

There was also a cookbook in the pipeline and this pleased Dave endlessly. Working and earning made him feel normal again and I couldn't have been more proud of him when he later opened up a box of freshly printed copies of *Ultimate Comfort Food* bearing their names. What an achievement.

In August 2023 between filming legs and treatment days, I managed to fulfil the promise I'd made to Dave when he first got ill and took him back to Lake Geneva. He made the online booking for hotels, crossings and stops, and I drove all the way there, returning to the same room in the Grand Hôtel du Lac in Vevey overlooking the lake where we'd first stayed back in 2018. We'd also returned the following year with some of Dave's brethren from the Water Rats to visit Charlie Chaplin's house and museum.

This time was the most special and we appreciated every second of being there together. With short strolls on the promenade to see the Fork of Vevey (an eight-metre tall, stainless-steel fork which stands on the shore of Lake Geneva), relaxing on benches, watching people pedalling on the water and dining at the Buddha Bar, we found a serenity that was very much needed.

I'm so glad we had that time because towards the end of October, things started to change. Dave seemed increasingly tired and his blood results were not great. Nevertheless, he managed to finish the TV series and then work on a Christmas special, which ended with a dinner for some of our friends and contributors to the show as well as the medical team caring for him at the hospital.

My man looked shattered. He never spoke about it, but I could sense he was slowly giving up. He painted a mask of bravery on his lovely face and hid his true feelings behind smiles ... but as his wife and soulmate, I could see it.

I could feel it.

I almost feel guilty admitting that I've still not watched that final award-winning series because I'm not sure I could bear it. Most people wouldn't notice or realise the significance, but Dave was far more poorly than he let on publicly at that point – I know I'd recognise a look on his face, a slight wince in the way he moved or steadied his balance, and I don't want to be reminded of his struggle.

As soon as he finished the voiceovers for *Go West* I took him away to Tenerife for a week in the sun. I knew if we stayed at home he would find it difficult as the realisation that his working days were over sank in. I worried that the melancholy would make things progress more quickly, and so I pushed for one more experience with him, one more adventure to take us away from what we knew was coming.

He took some convincing because the trip meant taking a flight and Dave was quite understandably scared of airports, but when we got to the island, he promptly relaxed. We did very little else that week other than read, rest, eat and swim. There was no one to bother us, no distractions or other commitments, just us being together. Dave's insatiable appetite for reading was still there – this was a man who would often have several books on the go at once. He loved thrillers by John Grisham and Ian Rankin but also enjoyed getting stuck into non-fiction where he could learn about history and people and cultures.

He loved our trip to Tenerife so much, he booked another at the same place for that coming Christmas, this time for the whole family, Sergiu, Iza and their partners. Maybe it was a valiant attempt to delay the inevitable or perhaps it was a superhuman effort to make me happy and get another break into the bank of memories. Whatever the motivation, I did my best to hide my fears and go along with his plans, hoping for the strength to go through with whatever he wanted.

But that last family trip was not to be. When I woke up on the morning of 22 December, the day we were due to fly out, I turned my head in Dave's direction and knew instantly we were not going anywhere apart from to the hospital. I could see the disappointment in his eyes and knew he felt he was letting me down.

'Darling,' I said, 'you're not well. Please don't feel bad.'

I put him in the car and we headed straight to the hospital where we spent the whole day having tests, none of which gave us good news. The kids had already flown by that point and we told them to stay in Tenerife and make the most of the holiday even though we were unable to join them. But that Christmas was not an easy one.

The last Christmas.

The last weeks of our life together.

The last desperate hopes vanishing with every breath.

* * *

Whether death comes suddenly or after a long journey of illness there's trauma for the people left behind. For the surviving partner and family, the pain of loss brings the same whys and what ifs, the same anger, despair, sorrow and guilt, all those daggers stabbing at the heart and tormenting the mind.

Perhaps having the time to say your goodbyes can help with so-called closure and therefore bring about some sense of peace, but there's little comfort in that when you have to witness your loved one gradually shrinking, their wits and spirit dissolving before your eyes. The sadness and powerlessness I felt while nursing Dave during his final days are indescribable. Watching his vitality slowly disappear, the fire in his eyes turning to tiredness, his brilliance being blunted by medication, his body shrivelling and the hope fading away … until there was no hope left at all.

Just pain, pills and drips to manage.

After being in and out of hospital over Christmas, New Year and over the first week of 2024, Dave was allowed home where I looked after him, supported by district nurses, the odd visit from the GP and an army of friends and family who made sure I was never alone. I guess some of my educated instincts kicked in because subconsciously I knew this moment was bigger than me. I had the power to ask for help and help duly arrived.

Dr Dave, whose daughter Amy was heavily pregnant at the time, travelled down from Aberdeenshire every other week, sometimes driving through the night or battling through train strikes to do so. That man is a hero. His beautiful grandson was born a couple of weeks after Dave died and they named him Harris David.

I invited old friends to come and visit so they'd have a chance to say their goodbyes. We had people in the house all the time.

Sergiu and Iza. Their partners, Mara and Emilio.

Simon.

Milly, Jacqui and Cath.

Claire and Bridget.

Nic and Tash.

Reverend Richard.

All these wonderful humans helping us during the most harrowing time of our life.

On autopilot, I busied myself with the everyday jobs that needed doing. I made sure there was wood by the fireplace and that the fire was always roaring in Dave's favourite room with all his antiques. I'd take Teddy out for walks. Clinging on to those mundane tasks as if my life depended on them.

Dave was eating less and less every day, wasting away, and I could do nothing but cry in despair and frustration at my limited abilities to make things better. Sometimes he'd tell me he fancied a McDonald's so I'd drive a few miles to fetch one, only to watch him push the plate away when I returned.

He was drifting in and out of sleep and needed increasing pain medication when awake. The desperation and confusion over what to do and how to handle it was overwhelming. I had no say in what went on, it just happened and I bore witness to it.

I didn't eat because my body didn't need or accept any food. At times I was barely breathing. I didn't feel anything beyond despair and a dull pain in my whole body. Everything felt surreal. The surreal imminence of death.

The finality of it.

And the awareness that my life would change in one moment whether I wanted it to or not. For two years I'd watched Dave die – every day a little bit more – hoping with all my will for a different outcome while also preparing myself for the worst.

As he took his last breaths, each one of them deepening the anguish inside of me, I tried to breathe for him, thinking maybe it would help him.

And then … silence.

The silence that comes after the final breath is simultaneously the worst pain and the most holy moment, because it signifies such profound and irreversible change. Everything after that is different. You're not the same person and never will be again. How can one breath change your life so much? As much as I hate the word with a passion, one breath made me a widow.

One breath.

One moment.

And there's no 'us' anymore. Just me.

The Recipes

2 February 2025

The wood burner in our kitchen crackles as I settle on the sofa with my laptop. I have emails to send out for the fast-approaching Dave Day 2 – there's a lot for me and the ambitious team to organise following the huge success of the first event last June.

Busy. It feels good to be busy.

This kitchen was one of the big selling points of the house for Dave, with its open space, bespoke units, granite work surfaces and four-oven AGA. Sadly, he didn't get the chance to enjoy it half as much as he should have, but he's still everywhere in it. His pots, pans and crockery collection are here on the open shelving as well as his set of crystal champagne coupes we bought at The Ritz on one of our special weekend treats and where the head chef John Williams had served up a meal beyond compare.

There's also his ever-expanding spice rack which, over the years, became a full-blown pantry. A museum of spice!

Dave couldn't go anywhere without picking up a few more samples of this or that – I remember he went so wild in a food market in Istanbul with all the smells, colours and textures that we had to pay for an extra checked-in bag just to get his new spices on the flight home.

When he came back from filming *The Hairy Bikers' Asian Adventure* in the Far East, he brought home jars of dried bugs which we would just look at from time to time, mainly in horror. He never used them, he was just so curious having seen people cooking with them, so they became part of his treasure trove.

Another time he returned from Mexico with a big bag of dried chillies, which he would often dip into if he wanted to add an extra kick to a dish. Until, that is, he discovered that a naughty house mouse had chewed through the bag, eaten his precious Mexican chillies and left only a few dried seeds behind. Poor Dave was bereft for days.

Over in the far corner of the kitchen is a bookcase that is home to his hundreds of recipe books, cookery magazines and handwritten notebooks, all collected from travels around the country and the world. Every cuisine you could think of is covered here. Most of them have stained pages, yellowed by oils or turmeric or splattered by spilt coffee and many still carry his fingerprints in some spice mix, a permanent reminder of his mad, messy days in the kitchen. He never stopped looking out for new flavours, new combinations, new ways of cooking different foods.

Dave and Me

'Eat that and you'll live forever!' he'd say as he served up a dish he'd spent hours concocting.

I put the laptop to one side and walk over to the bookcase, suddenly drawn to it. There are books here by all the greats: Marco Pierre White, Keith Floyd who Dave adored, Delia Smith. There are quite a few by James Martin, another chef Dave had a lot of time for, both professionally and personally. Whenever the Bikers were doing festivals at the same time as James, they'd crash each other's stage which gave the crowds a huge amount of pleasure.

Dave always raved about doing James's *Saturday Kitchen*; he got such a buzz from being live on TV and he loved it when there were spicy stories to tell.

Like when Dave and Si had to do the show's famous Omelette Challenge where celeb chefs are set the task of making a three-egg omelette as quickly as possible. Dave was determined to win and had put himself on an intensive training regime, getting through dozens of eggs at home the week before while I timed him with a stopwatch. But when it came to the live show it didn't quite go according to plan and he found that he couldn't break the eggs. Dave thought he was going mad until he realised Simon had hard boiled them all earlier to stitch him up.

Ah, here are a couple of titles by Mary Berry – Dave particularly admired her simple and realistic cooking methods – and a number by Rick Stein. Dave appreciated Rick's gentle way of approaching the food and cultures he was visiting.

There are a few very personal, handwritten cookbooks he received from people who wanted him to have them, gifting their late mother's old recipes to a person they knew would truly appreciate them. Pieces of history.

'Lil,' he'd say, 'I can feel what that person was feeling when they wrote this recipe inherited from their aunt ... and leaving it as a legacy for their family. This is social history!'

I flick through some of the books and see Dave's distinctive handwriting in notes scribbled in the margins, the bent corners and ripped pages all testament to a life full of flavour and fun. The kitchen was his domain – his heaven – and I loved sitting with a glass of vino in my hand, watching him in action while we put the world to rights.

What's left after losing him? The kitchen is still here and his belongings are all in their place. I can still touch them, but they are soulless now.

What's left is only the grief that I'm learning how to metabolise, to integrate and move forward with.

'Grief turns out to be a place none of us know until we reach it,' wrote Joan Didion in her memoir *The Year of Magical Thinking* documenting the 12 months following the sudden death of her husband, John Gregory Dunne. It's a quote that strikes a chord because it captures the intensely personal and unpredictable nature of grief. It is about much more than loss and so much more than a mere *feeling* ... it is a state of being and a force with the power to reshape all it touches.

Dave and Me

And I don't own this grief by myself. Many people around me were deeply affected by what happened to Dave during his illness and his passing, beautiful people who I relied on and who relied on me. My son and daughter lost their anchor, too ... their father figure, role model, friend and confidant. They would call Dave and have long conversations with him far more than they would with me – he always brought the fun and took a positive attitude to whatever was going on in their lives. My role, as mum, was more 'the voice of reason'. Dave was the playmate who would shuffle the cards and let them pick the game.

As a family we were deeply connected, every life moment – big or small – was shared and Dave was so proud of us as a unit, and of Sergiu and Iza individually.

My perception of everything changes and evolves depending on the filters or triggers of the day. Some days I view things with pain and anger, other days it's with calmness or acceptance. I write down my thoughts and feelings only to read them back later and find myself realigning everything from a different perspective entirely. This is all part of something I'm learning about in real time as I live it.

It is a complex and personal journey with no recipe or guidebook on how to handle it 'properly'. One of the most poignant descriptions I've come across is the pearl analogy. Pearls form when grains of sand or a parasite enters the shell of an oyster, damaging the fragile flesh. As a defence mechanism, the oyster produces layers of nacre (also known as mother-of-pearl), encasing the intruder which, over time, turns it into a beautiful pearl. I see this as being similar to how grief affects us.

It is always going to be there. But if we surround it with layers of tears, experience, feelings and colour, we can grow around it. As we become stronger, the grief becomes integrated and it makes us more resilient people, richer in feelings, deeper in understanding, wiser and more generous with others.

And in the end, just like the pearl, we emerge as something more beautiful than before.

Chapter Twelve

Dave Day

My throat is as dry as Gandhi's flip-flops!

The days after Dave left us were a chaotic mix of confusion, pain, heaviness and emptiness. Family and friends kept each other company in Dave's favourite room, talking about him, crying, laughing, feeling him all around us.

It had happened and it was final. There was nothing I, or any of us, could do about it.

No turning back from this.

It wasn't that I refused to accept it, I just couldn't yet fathom the magnitude of what it all meant and was unable to articulate how I felt. There was an astounding outpouring of love and support from the public and I found some solace reading through the countless messages people I'd never met had taken the time to send me. Many were asking if there was a way they could show how much he had meant to them.

Was there any scope for some kind of tribute or day of celebration?

So this was something I was already mulling over on the day of the funeral when I floated the idea of organising a ride in Dave's memory to some friends, including Jason 'Woody' Woodcock who we'd first met through the Sons of Royalty charity motorcycle rides. Woody is a mad biker, ex-military police and a beautiful friend, generous with his time and always there when he is needed. I've seen him in action saving lives and have heard stories of his incredible bravery.

'Just say when and we'll do it,' he said.

It was as simple as that at the start, although I could never have imagined it would become what it did.

We found Simon, pulling him into our group conversation for his thoughts and quickly settled on the date of Saturday, 8 June 2024. Others joined the discussion and it started to gain legs. Or, rather, wheels! Paul, a solicitor friend from Barrow, overheard us talking and he said, 'I see something growing here ... you're peppering it, you're sprinkling it and it's going to keep on growing.'

Which is exactly what happened. Word spread rapidly and by the following day we had a Facebook account inviting people to register if they wanted to take part in what was going to be a 300-mile ride from London to Barrow in memory of Dave.

Within 24 hours of that we had a couple of hundred signed up, which would turn out to be just the tip of a very large iceberg. We also opened a donations page, setting a £5,000 target to raise money to be split between the NSPCC, Childline and the Institute of Cancer Research. We hit that target in a matter of days, so we raised it again. And then again. In the end we would go on to raise over £130,000.

The power of Dave Myers.

The phrase 'I'm having a Dave Day' came from one of the social media messages. This person wrote:

The word 'Dave' should be the new adjective when it comes to expressing joy, happiness and a lust for life … Just imagine people saying: 'I've had a real Dave day today, it's going great and I feel so Dave today!'

It was perfect and so we adopted it for the ride. I wish I could remember who wrote it so I can credit them properly. I still hope they might get back in touch.

Over the next few weeks, supported by Woody and many other friends, I threw my all into organising Dave Day. There was an awful lot to arrange in a short space of time, but we were all determined to make this happen, knowing it was something that would bring joy to a lot of people.

Woody was the capable person dealing with the ride itself, organising the logistics for the day, and we decided it would start in the morning at the Ace Café in northwest London, right by the North Circular, then make its way up the country, heading through Oxford, Birmingham and along the M6 before finishing in Barrow-in-Furness that evening where there would be a huge party.

By 8 June, we had around 2,000 people registered to take part in the ride, which we thought was a brilliant number. However, many more than that turned up on the day and, led by Woody and Si, the convoy left London at 8am sharp. Bikers joined the throng at every stop along the route. They picked up a few thousand at Oxford Services on the M40 and thousands more still at the National Motorcycle Museum in Birmingham on the M42.

I was nervously waiting for them with Si's partner, Jenny, Iza and her partner, Emilio, further north at Knutsford Services, ready to jump on the back of Woody's bike for the remainder of the journey to Barrow. Jenny and I had arrived at 10 am, a fair bit before the convoy was due, and there were only seven or eight bikes waiting with us at first. But over the next two hours there was a trickle, then a stream and in the end a flood of bikes to the area until the whole place was teeming with riders.

By the time Si, Woody and the entourage reached Knutsford, there were around 7,000 of us there to greet them, motorbikes and people everywhere. It's hard to describe what I was feeling, but I knew something amazing, something unbelievable, something far bigger than any of us was happening. It was like a unified field of camaraderie, friendship, empathy and sympathy engulfing everybody present, touching hearts and bringing tears to our eyes.

When I saw Si, he was crying and he took me in his arms while the crowd surrounded us.

'We've done it!' I said.

'Every bridge, Lil,' replied Si. 'There were people on every bridge for your man.'

Everyone was crying with us and we felt the collective love holding us in those moments. And then I climbed on the back of Woody's bike, Jenny got on the back of Si's and we set off from Knutsford, leading this sea of riders, many of them wearing Dave-style Hawaiian shirts over their biking gear. What a glorious spectacle.

The police closed that section of the northbound M6 to allow every bike to exit the services together and we were waved off by hundreds of well-wishers standing on the bridge above while cars heading south on the other side of the motorway beeped their horns in solidarity.

The last stop before Barrow was Burton-in-Kendal Services where thousands more bikes were waiting to join us for the final leg, but about five miles before we arrived, the police put out a message that there wasn't going to be enough room for us to enter and that we'd have to pass by. This caused a mild panic for Woody, who knew that many bikers needed fuel (and a toilet break!), so the police officer who had been escorting us sped on ahead and organised a corridor – a parting of the ways – just wide enough for our bikes to get through.

Among those waiting for us there was Dr Dave, who had ridden a rented bike from Aberdeenshire to join the party, and after a short break for Woody, Si, plus a few other bikes who had managed to squeeze in while the rest of the convoy hung back, we were back on the road again, joined by the thousands who had waited for us in Burton-in-Kendal.

On the final 30 miles into Barrow, there were people along every inch of that roadside. It was as beautiful as it was humbling and it felt like we were flying.

We eventually rode into Dave's beloved hometown at four o'clock in the afternoon to a hero's welcome, and the bikes behind us continued arriving until half past seven – that's how huge it was. Even the normally gloomy Barrow weather, which I'd struggled to adapt to when we lived there years before, came through for us. The sun shone all day long – just 24 hours before it had been chucking it down, so I can only believe that Dave somehow arranged all that.

But this was a day when humanity shone, too.

Si, Woody and I addressed the thousands gathered outside the town hall where the local authorities had built us a stage and we thanked everybody for their support and involvement. The tears flowed again as I was presented with a posthumous Freedom of the Town for Dave while local artists played live music.

Later that evening, the Barrow Raiders rugby club hosted a rock concert at their stadium, Craven Park, where musicians – many of them friends – performed for free to be part of this special celebration. The band Massive Wagons headlined with Susie Webb, Maiden Cumbria, Blue Nation and Thunder's Luke Morley also on the bill.

A very generous lady called Trish donated her late husband's motorbike to be auctioned, which raised even more for our charities.

A Dave Day indeed!

I spoke to so many people that day who had found something in his story to connect with. Some were going through cancer themselves, others were grieving loved ones and had not yet found a way to deal with their loss. They sobbed as they told me about their journeys, their pain, their losses and how they'd found this event to be a positive outlet for their emotions.

Somebody sent me a message afterwards saying they'd been bereaved in lockdown when it had not been possible to attend funerals. On Dave Day, they had discovered the closure they'd been searching for.

I heard later about an older gentleman who was quite sick and in a wheelchair, unable to get out of the house. His son had put a post on the Dave Day social pages about how much his father would have loved to see the parade and so hundreds of bikers took a ride past his house where he'd cheered them on from his chair. What a kind and very human gesture and so typical of the community Dave loved so much.

Dave Day meant a lot of things for a lot of people, which was such an unexpected bonus. The whole event was powered by kindness and the very best of people who were so generous with their time, efforts, resources and talents, whether that was donating money or sponsorship, marshalling the route, taking part in the ride itself, helping to organise licences, performing for free or providing sarnies and water for the bikers.

What I took away from this unparalleled event can't be expressed in words.

THE LOVE.

I knew Dave and Si were in the public's hearts, but I never thought his passing would open such a huge expression of love for him and for what he represented.

THE LIFE.

Dave was a family man, a celebrity, a chef, a biker, a writer, a makeup artist. An ordinary Barrow lad doing extraordinary things and this was inspirational for so many.

THE FRIENDSHIP.

What Dave and Si had on the screen and in real life truly resonated.

THE RIDE.

It brought togetherness in the biking community in a way not many had seen before. Not to mention the inspiration it gave to the thousands of spectators.

THE COMMUNITY.

People came together in the most inclusive and uplifting way. Everyone who made this happen is an incredible human being and deserves praise over and over again.

THE JOURNEY.

Cancer touches so many lives and Dave Day gave people an outlet for their pain, grief and loss.

We all, as a collective, lived something unique, basking in a big halo of love, unity, friendship and positivity. Together we made history.

If you made a banner, decorated your shop front, covered the potholes in the road (that did make me laugh), stood on a bridge on the motorway to give us a Dave wave, came to meet us in the petrol stations or lined the streets as we pulled into town: from the bottom of my heart, thank you.

Weeks after the event, a mum sent me a message to tell me that her five-year-old daughter had said, 'Mummy, I can't stop waving at motorbikes because it makes me smile.' I thought that was wonderful.

There was magic on Dave Day.

We even had people fall in love. Laura from Barrow got in touch to say she'd met her soulmate, who was one of the riders. He's since moved from the Midlands up to Cumbria to be with her and they're very happy together. All these little sprinkles of beauty. The synchronicities making everything worthwhile.

Many people were inspired to take up motorcycling themselves, myself included! I've been learning ever since and plan to have my biking licence in time for Dave Day 2 in 2025 so I can ride on my own. It wasn't ever something I'd considered doing before because I was always happy being a pillion, but I think Dave's little gremlin has found a new home on my shoulder and it's pushed me into it. I've had nothing but encouragement from the biking community since I started my lessons, and when I posted on social media about having fallen a few times, hundreds of them sent messages urging me to continue and not to give up. They are an astonishingly kind group of people.

Did Dave ever know how much he was loved? He and Si were conscious of the fact that for so many years they were part of people's lives and in their living rooms. People considered them friends and I'd seen that numerous times when Dave was approached in public, something he always appreciated. But would he ever have imagined that something like this could be organised in his name? I don't think so.

For me, it reinforced that I was not alone in my grief. That has helped me start to learn to live without him, to bring out the best of what we had together and then carry that forward in a positive way.

I don't want to spend my life crying as a widow about time lost. I want to laugh and love and feel joy in my heart every day just like he did.

I want to – and I will – have Dave Days for the rest of my life.

Chapter Thirteen

Facing the Future

look at the blush on those snadgers!

Life stood still when I lost Dave. Even now it seems desolate and sad, although at times over the last year it's also felt as if I've been caught in a continuous race. I don't even know why I've been racing … probably some kind of an attempt to deflect pockets of grief. Grief not only for the loss of my husband, but also for what could have been and now never will.

Learning how to live with grief is not a linear process and neither is the process of understanding your limits, your resources, your strengths and weaknesses.

There have been moments when, not yet understanding my powers, I reached exhaustion, when my batteries have been so depleted that my body physically ached from the tiredness and my mind has gone completely blank. We can't operate when we are deprived of energy like this and it's something I have to remind myself repeatedly. I need to make sure to keep my cup full which means taking plenty of

279

rest and regular exercise, eating well and surrounding myself with good people.

I have had to be very careful not to give in to the overwhelming temptation to hide away on my own. It would be so easy to retreat to a dark place where I'd survive only on memories, be devoid of ambition and make zero attempt to fill this life, now empty of Dave, with anything that is not him. I'd quite easily bed in and abandon myself to pain and self-pity, allowing the 'why him?' and 'why me?' questions to rage through my head, becoming immobilised by the fear of 'what next?'

What next?

It doesn't matter how much I want to hang on to the person I was before Dave died; that version of me no longer exists. I'm more serious, less vibrant. I used to wear colourful clothes but for some reason I don't fancy them anymore. Maybe that will change again, maybe not – perhaps that's a side of me that is gone forever.

I know I must redefine my identity and figure out who I am without him, but it all feels so alien to me because my sense of self was so wrapped up in him and still is.

Everything I am is also him.

Everything I do is for us both.

Everything I have is ours.

Recovering a sense of joy and meaning after a traumatic event is a gradual and deeply personal process. How do you accept, readjust and reinvent yourself in these circumstances? How do you fill the void, reorientate, refocus and find purpose again?

And yet, healing *is* possible and there *are* ways to begin gently moving towards a fulfilled life once more.

You're not the same person as before and that invites changed behaviour, habits and connections. Embrace that, don't be afraid. But all in good time and at your own pace. Allow yourself time, and remember that time is not always the healer, but what you do with your time can help you heal. It's also crucial to remember that no two individuals' reactions to trauma are the same, so there's little point in comparing your progress to anyone else's. Allow yourself space and give yourself permission to feel, without judgement, whatever comes up, whether that's sadness, anger, longing or confusion.

Take every little win along the way, every glimmer, and celebrate them – they are your first steps towards a glimpse of happiness. Start a new hobby, something to engage the brain. Trying something new, however small, can help reawaken curiosity and even excitement over time.

Redefine what 'normality' is to you, and then slowly step into that new version. Connect to people, whether they've been in your life for a while, have slipped off your radar, or they're new attachments altogether. Accept the support when it's offered and don't be afraid to ask for it when you need it. These past months I've had a lot of help, for which I'm eternally grateful.

And on the flip side of that, if you know somebody who is going through a bereavement or any other major life event, don't just ask, 'Can I help?' Instead, offer to do something specific.

Can I pick your child up from school?

Can I bring you some bread and milk?

Can I drive you to an appointment?

Let me take you for a coffee.

It is much easier to accept support when the approach is not a vague one.

These are all steps I've taken and which have helped me pull myself up and get out into the light.

I have also had to learn to forgive myself for many things I thought I'd done or not done. It's often hard to silence that pesky inner judge who is always present, ready to berate us for things that were beyond our control, making us doubt ourselves for decisions we can't change.

Could have, would have, should have.

Cancelling out that noise is hard but it's part of the journey to find peace and accept ourselves for the good and bad, for our strengths and our flaws. For me, it's also been about letting go of my guilt that his illness happened on my watch and my attachment to an idea of a future he's not physically part of. And then making space for something new and unfamiliar.

These are all conscious decisions.

When life crumbles we can become stuck in a very painful place where anger, self-pity and bitterness rule the roost.

Or we can view it as a new beginning, as harsh as that might sound or seem. This is scary at first because it's unknown territory and requires us to put the work in to rediscover who we are, to rebuild ourselves in ways we hadn't ever considered, to dig deep and uncover inner strength we never knew we had. If you find yourself in such a situation right now, please know that you're braver than you believe, stronger than you seem and smarter than you think.

It's incredibly daunting, especially when life quietens and you're left to figure out how to navigate the journey ahead without a partner to share all the pleasures and the challenges. You no longer have your person to confer with or to lean on for advice; suddenly, you're on your own and it's down to you to make all the decisions.

But I have had to decide between my life being a continuous bereavement journey or becoming what Dave always taught me to be: a go-getter, someone who is living life fearlessly.

I have made that choice.

There is always grief to push through, but I won't let that hold me back or make me ill because I know Dave wouldn't want that for me. I will make his impact on my life meaningful by carrying on having adventures and experiencing life with him in my heart.

I am allowing this energy to push me in directions I never thought I would take and it's changing the way I see the world. My life doesn't have to shrink because Dave is not here; instead it can open up new opportunities to embrace.

I'm riding a motorbike.

I'm writing this book.

At the beginning of 2025 I took a solo trip to South Africa which was emotionally and spiritually uplifting and has made me hungry for more. We always spoke about going to Australia at some point – Dave had never been and it was on his To Do list, so now I will do that for us both. Argentina, too. Dave was enthralled by the country when he filmed over there and it was a place we planned to visit together. I loved hearing his stories about how he and Si had biked all the way down through Patagonia in the far south to watch the penguins and whales.

Looks like I'll have to go on my own … and I will.

I'm happy to see the world for him and to continue going to the magical places he would have been exploring had he lived.

I'm living now for him as well.

I talk to him all the time and feel his presence everywhere. Just recently I was chatting to another lady who had lost her husband and she asked me how I was managing to carry on. 'Well, I can feel his hand resting on my shoulder now,' I replied. And I really could. It was physical and real, reassuring and familiar.

The more I do things on my own, the braver I become. In November 2024, nine months after Dave passed, I attended the Grand Order of the Water Rats annual ball alone in his honour where they took a moment to pay tribute to him and other lost brethren. His picture came up on the screen to the applause of everybody in the room – his peers in the entertainment industry – which felt very special to be part of.

In February 2025, I went up on stage at London's Hilton on Park Lane to accept, along with Si, a TV Choice Award for Best Food Show, given to the team for the *Go West* series. An emotional night, and for Si too given that it was probably the last time there would be an occasion like this for the Bikers.

Finding my feet in this unfamiliar landscape is taking time because my life revolved around him. We women tend to do that, don't we? As wives, mums and carers, we can lose our identities while looking after the people around us. We don't remember who we are very often and we forget to live for ourselves.

In the years I was with Dave, entangled in his energy and swept along with his lust for life, I didn't take time to press pause and be curious about who I was. He was enough for me; he was the container for my universe and what he offered me was exciting and beautiful. But it would be deeply unfair of me to project this on Dave. I've been my own master before and I'm capable of managing after. He would *hate* to think I had no direction, that I was frozen in time, grieving for him, not knowing which way to turn.

And so, I'm on this path to becoming a new version of myself. I'm learning while I travel, sometimes taking big strides, other times just baby steps, leaving baggage behind as I go. It's a complex and unwieldy journey and, believe me,

I have questioned whether it is too soon even to consider moving on.

How can I move on from this exhilarating, out-of-the-ordinary life I shared with such an exceptional man? How is that possible when he is still everywhere and in everything around me?

But I know the answer now and it's very simple. I have been walking through grief with love in my heart and what that taught me is that I haven't lost myself, I have found a deeper me.

I can do it because I will move forward *with* him. I'm choosing to write my own narrative and to see this as a new start and I'm taking Dave with me, discovering who I am as I go.

He will always be part of me – I am me because of him – but it is time to know myself again. For Dave.

For both of us.

A Letter to Dave

My darling,

We once had the world at our feet and were drinking love potion in our cups every day while navigating through our time together. We loved with such intensity and so much fun that it was enough to last ten lifetimes. I'm now living with the empty space you left behind, thanking every moment for the cups we drank together, for they are keeping my heart full and my system alive.

I came into this world on the 28th day of a month and you chose to leave it on a 28th day. A beginning and an end shaping our existence, with a whole life happening in between. How privileged were we to have met and shared 20 years of togetherness in the most meaningful way. Your last 20 years. The best!

There will be milestones on my path forward, Christmases without your presents, anniversaries in your absence, birthdays to celebrate and memories to honour. All with you in my heart, all picturing you smiling and approving of what is going on. Feeling your presence and your light, for you are holding the torch showing my path ahead and I will follow it with gratitude.

Our lives change constantly, no matter how much we want to hang on to people, things or moments, and the only control we have is in how we react to change. You took the changes in your life and rode your bike for miles and miles, showing us all how to get on with things, even in the deepest, darkest hours. What a hero.

You inspired this book. It was such a joy to see the words forming phrases, the phrases describing our experiences and bringing feelings to the surface. Every page was taking shape under my fingertips in such a meaningful way. It was a pleasure to bring to light your life behind the camera, to give voice to your brilliance and expose your exuberance. It made me feel closer to you, understand you better and reframe my grief so I can carry it with integrity and love.

And just as you inspired me, I hope this book can inspire others. There's more to life than just surviving – life needs to be lived with wonder, happiness and freedom. We are the ones who need to give ourselves permission to do so, to see the beauty in every flower and every bright star in the night sky.

I can only express my gratitude for being part of your extraordinary journey and for having you as such a wonderful part of me. You made me trust that this life is worth living in love, and in full.

And for that, I'm eternally grateful.

With love,
 Your Lil

Acknowledgements

This book could not have happened without the trust and help my team has given me, or without the love my friends and family have surrounded me with.

Si King, you have been a constant in our life from day one, as a friend and as a business partner. You must have been experiencing the same sadness and helplessness as me in the last couple of years of Dave's life, watching him go through his illness. Thank you for all these years of friendship and support.

To my dear Easton friends, you know what you've done for Dave and me over the years!

My Dave Day team: Woody, Adele, Nicola, Wendy, Paul, Whitney, Lisa, the marshals and volunteers … You selflessly gave your time, knowledge and resources for free to bring this event to the public. You rock!

To my literary agent, Amanda Harris, who believed in this book from the beginning – a huge thank-you for steering my steps in the right direction and making things happen!

To my publishers, the wonderful team at Ebury, thank you for taking this idea and running with it! From the very first call with Charlotte Hardman, who deserves my deepest gratitude, the whole process has been tremendous for me. You've all made this book happen in a relatively short space of time, which took a huge effort, and you had faith that it would bring joy to the readers. Beth, you helped me shape my thoughts, thank you! Jasmin, Lucy, Ellenor, thank you for organising every aspect of moving this book in the right direction. Honestly, I feel like I've had the best team possible to bring this story to the readers.

And I want to express gratitude to the people in my life I shall never forget:

The ones who listened when I had very little or nothing to say and had faith in me, knowing I'd find my voice.

The ones who stuck around when I might have tried to push them away.

The ones who helped me without asking for anything in return.

The ones who didn't let me settle for less than I deserved, even when I couldn't see clearly.

The ones who forgave me for my words or behaviour when I couldn't forgive myself.

The ones who celebrated my successes, big or small, when I didn't feel worthy of celebration.

The ones who were there when I felt small and invisible, and helped me build myself up and stand tall.

The ones who loved me when I didn't feel lovable.

The ones who apologised even when they didn't have to.

Dave and Me

The ones who didn't just say they cared but showed it.

The ones who were there for me even when I couldn't ask for help.

You all know who you are because you've helped me go through my deep valley and become stronger.

With gratitude,
    Lili